Praise for *The Vegetarian Myth*

The Vegetarian Myth is one of the most important books people, masses of them, can read, as we try with all our might, intelligence, skill, hope, dream and memory, to turn the disastrous course the planet is on. It's a wonderful book, full of thoughtful, soulful teachings, and appropriate rage.
—**Alice Walker**

Anyone who has ever read a book on writing has come across the hackneyed piece of advice to cut open a vein and bleed on the page. Lierre Keith has come closer to literally doing that than almost any writer I've ever read. Not only does her passion for her subject bleed through in almost every sentence, she is a superb lyrical prose stylist. My book is dog eared, underlined and annotated from front to back – I can't remember anything I've read that has contained so many terrific lines.

And if you have or know anyone with a daughter who is contemplating going vegetarian, please make this book available. It could be the most important thing you ever do for the long-term mental and physical health of a young woman.
—**Dr. Michael Eades**, author of *Protein Power* and *The 6-Week Cure for the Middle-Aged Middle*

This book saved my life. Not only does *The Vegetarian Myth* make clear how we should be eating, but also how the dominant food system is killing the planet. This necessary book challenges many of the destructive myths we live by and offers us a way back into our bodies, and back into the fight to save the planet.
—**Derrick Jensen**, author of *Endgame* and *A Language Older Than Words*

Everyone interested in healthy eating should be grateful to Lierre Keith. Her book will help many seekers to avoid the lesson she had to learn through bitter experience.
—**Sally Fallon Morell**, President, The Weston A. Price Foundation

What I thought would be a book filled with disgruntled accounts of a has-been vegetarian justifying the excuse to pig out on double cheeseburgers again, was actually a well-researched, statistically sound discussion of agriculture and its effects on land, society, animals, and the relationship between all three. For those who insist on one way versus another, *The Vegetarian Myth* presents us with enough information to wisely weigh whatever we choose to put on our plates.

—**Olupero R. Aiyenimelo**, FeministReview.org

Lierre Keith has written a compelling tale of her own near self-destruction from a vegan diet and a broadside against its being perpetrated upon or adopted by any other victims. She has converted 20 years of pain and suffering, and permanent damage to her health into a galvanizing passion to demolish the myth that she believes underpins the worldview of most who adopt vegan diet: "I want to eat without killing." You can't, she says, and if you try you'll die.

Keith has transmuted her anger and seasoned it well with a self-reflective humor that sweeps us along this road to recovery from a scorched earth. As I read her description of her first meat meal in 20 years (a can of tuna eaten reluctantly with a plastic fork), I found myself in tears. Ten years recovering from a quarter century of vegetarian folly myself, I knew the shattering epiphany she experienced with that first bite—coming home to the truth of her body, and of life itself.

—**Peter Bane**, *Permaculture Activist*

Everyone who eats should read this book. Everyone who eats vegetarian should memorize it. This is the single most important book I've ever read on diet, agriculture, and ecology. And as a farmer and ex-vegan, that's saying a lot.

—**Aric McBay**, author of *What We Leave Behind* and *Peak Oil Survival*

The Vegetarian Myth puts together in coherent and passionate form all the arguments about meat and agriculture that have been running around in my head for fifteen years. It's not easy to transmute outrage and pain into something so full of love and wonder, but Lierre Keith has done it beautifully.

—**Toby Hemenway**, author of *Gaia's Garden: A Guide to Home-Scale Permaculture*

The Vegetarian Myth

food, justice, and sustainability

Lierre Keith

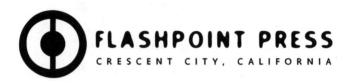

FLASHPOINT PRESS
CRESCENT CITY, CALIFORNIA

PM PRESS
P.O. BOX 23912, OAKLAND, CA 94623
WWW.PMPRESS.ORG

Also by Lierre Keith:

Conditions of War

Skyler Gabriel

Also from Flashpoint Press:

Now This War Has Two Sides
A spoken word CD set by Derrick Jensen

Lives Less Valuable
A novel by Derrick Jensen

Songs of the Dead
A novel by Derrick Jensen

How Shall I Live My Life?
Interviews by Derrick Jensen

The Day Philosophy Died
A Novel by Casey Maddox

To Annemarie Monahan, one of my favourite animals,

and

in memory of Terry Lotz.

Flashpoint Press
PO Box 903
Crescent City, CA 95531
www.flashpointpress.com

PM Press
PO Box 23912
Oakland, CA 94623
www.pmpress.org

Library of Congress Control Number:
2009921671

Book design by Aric McBay

Printed in the USA on recycled paper

9 7 8 1 6 0 4 8 6 0 8 0 1

Contents

CHAPTER 1
Why This Book?

This was not an easy book to write. For many of you, it won't be an easy book to read. I know. I was a vegan for almost twenty years. I know the reasons that compelled me to embrace an extreme diet and they are honorable, ennobling even. Reasons like justice, compassion, a desperate and all-encompassing longing to set the world right. To save the planet—the last trees bearing witness to ages, the scraps of wilderness still nurturing fading species, silent in their fur and feathers. To protect the vulnerable, the voiceless. To feed the hungry. At the very least to refrain from participating in the horror of factory farming.

These political passions are born of a hunger so deep that it touches on the spiritual. Or they were for me, and they still are. I want my life to be a battle cry, a war zone, an arrow pointed and loosed into the heart of domination: patriarchy, imperialism, industrialization, every system of power and sadism. If the martial imagery alienates you, I can rephrase it. I want my life—my body—to be a place where the earth is cherished, not devoured; where the sadist is granted no quarter; where the violence stops. And I want eating—the first nurturance—to be an act that sustains instead of kills.

This book is written to further those passions, that hunger. It is not an attempt to mock the concept of animal rights or to sneer at the people who want a gentler world. Instead, this book is an effort to honor our deepest longings for a just world. And those longings—for compassion, for sustainability, for an equitable distribution of resources—are not served by the philosophy or practice of vegetarianism. We have been led astray. The vegetarian Pied Pipers have the best of intentions. I'll state right now what I'll be repeating later: everything they say about factory farming is true. It is cruel, wasteful, and destructive. Nothing in this book is meant to excuse or promote the practices of industrial food production on any level.

But the first mistake is in assuming that factory farming—a practice that is barely fifty years old—is the only way to raise animals. Their calculations on energy used, calories consumed, humans unfed, are all based on the notion that animals eat grain.

You can feed grain to animals, but it is not the diet for which they were designed. Grain didn't exist until humans domesticated annual grasses, at most 12,000 years ago, while aurochs, the wild progenitors of the domestic cow, were around for two million years before that. For most of human history, browsers and grazers haven't been in competition with humans. They ate what we couldn't eat—cellulose—and turned it into what we could—protein and fat. Grain will dramatically increase the growth rate of beef cattle (there's a reason for the expression "cornfed") and the milk production of dairy cows. It will also kill them. The delicate bacterial balance of a cow's rumen will go acid and turn septic. Chickens get fatty liver disease if fed grain exclusively, and they don't need any grain to survive. Sheep and goats, also ruminants, should really never touch the stuff.

This misunderstanding is born of ignorance, an ignorance that runs the length and breadth of the vegetarian myth, through the nature of agriculture and ending in the nature of life. We are urban industrialists, and we don't know the origins of our food. This includes vegetarians, despite their claims to the truth. It included me, too, for twenty years. Anyone who ate meat was in denial; only I had faced the facts. Certainly, most people who consume factory-farmed meat have never asked what died and how it died. But frankly, neither have most vegetarians.

The truth is that agriculture is the most destructive thing humans have done to the planet, and more of the same won't save us. The truth is that agriculture requires the wholesale destruction of entire ecosystems. The truth is also that life isn't possible without death, that no matter what you eat, someone has to die to feed you.

I want a full accounting, an accounting that goes way beyond what's dead on your plate. I'm asking about everything that died in the process, everything that was killed to get that food onto your plate. That's the more radical question, and it's the only question that will produce the truth. How many rivers were dammed and drained, how many prairies plowed and forests pulled down, how much topsoil turned to dust and blown into ghosts? I want to know about all the species—not just the individuals, but the entire species—the chinook, the bison, the grasshopper sparrows, the grey wolves. And I want more than just the number of dead and gone. I want them back.

Despite what you've been told, and despite the earnestness of the tellers, eating soybeans isn't going to bring them back. Ninety-eight percent of the American prairie is gone, turned into a monocrop of annual grains. Plough cropping in Canada has destroyed 99 percent of the original humus.[1] In fact, the disappearance of topsoil "rivals global warming as an environmental threat."[2] When the rainforest falls to beef, progressives are outraged, aware, ready to boycott. But our attachment to the vegetarian myth leaves us uneasy, silent, and ultimately immobilized when the culprit is wheat and the victim is the prairie. We embraced as an article of faith that vegetarianism was the way to salvation, for us, for the planet. How could it be destroying either?

We have to be willing to face the answer. What's looming in the shadows of our ignorance and denial is a critique of civilization itself. The starting point may be what we eat, but the end is an entire way of life, a global arrangement of power, and no small measure of personal attachment to it. I remember the day in fourth grade when Miss Fox wrote two words on the blackboard: *civilization* and *agriculture*. I remember because of the hush in her voice, the gravitas of her words, the explanation that was almost oratory. This was Important. And I understood. Everything that was good in human culture flowed from this point: all ease, grace, justice. Religion, science, medicine, art were born, and the endless struggle against starvation, disease, violence could be won, all because humans figured out how to grow their own food.

The reality is that agriculture has created a net loss for human rights and culture: slavery, imperialism, militarism, class divisions, chronic hunger, and disease. "The real problem, then, is not to explain why some people were slow to adopt agriculture but why anybody took it up at all, when it is so obviously beastly," writes Colin Tudge of The London School of Economics.[3] Agriculture has also been devastating to the other creatures with whom we share the earth, and ultimately to the life support systems of the planet itself. What is at stake is everything. If we want a sustainable world, we have to be willing to examine the power relations behind the foundational myth of our culture. Anything less and we will fail.

Questioning at that level is difficult for most people. In this case, the emotional struggle inherent in resisting any hegemony is compounded by our dependence on civilization, and on our individual helplessness to stop it. Most of us would have no chance of survival if the industrial infrastructure collapsed tomorrow. And our consciousness is equally impeded by our powerlessness. There is no Ten Simple Things list in the last chapter because, frankly, there aren't ten simple things that will save the earth. There is no personal solution. There is an interlocking web of hierarchical arrangements, vast systems of power that have to be confronted and dismantled. We can disagree about how best to do that, but do it we must if the earth is to have any chance of surviving.

In the end, all the fortitude in the world will be useless without enough information to chart a sustainable forward course, both personally and politically. One of my aims in writing this book is to provide that information. The vast majority of people in the US don't grow food, let alone hunt and gather it.[4] We have no way to judge how much death is embodied in a serving of salad, a bowl of fruit, a plate of beef. We live in urban environments, in the last whisper of forests, thousands of miles removed from the devastated rivers, prairies, wetlands, and the millions of creatures who died for our dinners. We don't even know what questions to ask to find out.

In his book *Long Life, Honey in the Heart*, Martin Pretchel writes of the Mayan people and their concept of *kas-limaal*, which translates roughly as "mutual indebtedness, mutual insparkedness."[5] "The knowledge that every animal, plant, person, wind, and season is indebted to the fruit of everything else is an adult knowledge. To get out of debt means you don't want to be part of life, and you don't want to grow into an adult," one of the elders explains to Pretchel.

The only way out of the vegetarian myth is through the pursuit of *kas-limaal*, of adult knowledge. This is a concept we need, especially those of us who are impassioned by injustice. I know I needed it. In the narrative of my life, the first bite of meat after my twenty year hiatus marks the end of my youth, the moment when I assumed the responsibilities of adulthood. It was the moment I stopped fighting the basic algebra of embodiment: for someone to live, someone else has to die. In that acceptance, with all its suffering and sorrow, is the ability to choose a different way, a better way.

The activist-farmers have a very different plan than the polemicist-writers to carry us from destruction to sustainability. The farmers are starting with completely different information. I've heard vegetarian activists claims that an acre of land can only support two chickens. Joel Salatin, one of the High Priests of sustainable farming and someone who actually raises chickens, puts that figure at 250 an acre.[6] Whom do you believe? How many of us know enough to even have an opinion? Frances Moore Lappé says it takes twelve to sixteen pounds of grain to make one pound of beef.[7] Meanwhile, Salatin raises cattle with no grain at all, rotating ruminants on perennial polycultures, building topsoil year by year. Inhabitants of urban industrial cultures have no point of contact with grain, chickens, cows, or, for that matter, with topsoil. We have no basis of experience to outweigh the arguments of political vegetarians. We have no idea what plants, animals, or soil eat, or how much. Which means we have no idea what we ourselves are eating.

Confronting the truth about factory farming—its torturous treatment of animals, its environmental toll—was for me at age sixteen an act of profound importance. I knew the earth was dying. It was a daily emergency I had lived against forever. I was born in 1964.

"Silent" and "spring" were inseparable: three syllables, not two words. Hell was here, in the oil refineries of northern New Jersey, the asphalt inferno of suburban sprawl, in the swelling tide of humans drowning the planet. I cried with Iron Eyes Cody, longed for his silent canoe and an unmolested continent of rivers and marshes, birds and fish. My brother and I would climb an ancient crabapple tree at the local park and dream about somehow buying a whole mountain. No people allowed, no discussion needed. Who would live there? Squirrels, was all I could come up with. Reader, don't laugh. Besides Bobby, our pet hamster, squirrels were the only animals I ever saw. My brother, well-socialized into masculinity, went on to torture insects and aim slingshots at sparrows. I became a vegan.

Yes, I was an overly sensitive child. My favorite song at five—and here you are allowed to laugh—was Mary Hopkin's *Those Were the Days*. What romantic, tragic past could I possibly have mourned at age five? But it was so sad, so exquisite; I would listen to the song over and over until I was exhausted from weeping.

Okay, it's funny. But I can't laugh at the pain I felt over my powerless witnessing of the destruction of my planet. That was real and it overwhelmed me. And the political vegetarians offered a compelling salve. With no understanding of the nature of agriculture, the nature of nature, or ultimately the nature of life, I had no way to know that however honorable their impulses, their prescription was a dead end into the same destruction I burned to stop.

Those impulses and ignorances are inherent to the vegetarian myth. For two years after I returned to eating meat, I was compelled to read vegan message boards online. I don't know why. I wasn't looking for a fight. I never posted anything myself. Lots of small, intense subcultures have cult-like elements, and veganism is no exception. Maybe the compulsion had to do with my own confusion—spiritual, political, personal. Maybe I was revisiting the site of an accident: this was where I had destroyed my body. Maybe I had questions and I wanted to see if I could hold my own against the answers that I had once held tight, answers that had felt righteous, but now felt empty. Maybe I don't know why. It left me anxious, angry, and desperate each time.

But one post marked a turning point. A vegan flushed out his idea to keep animals from being killed—not by humans, but by other animals. Someone should build a fence down the middle of the Serengeti, and divide the predators from the prey. Killing is wrong and no animals should ever have to die, so the big cats and wild canines would go on one side, while the wildebeests and zebras would live on the other. He knew the carnivores would be okay because they didn't need to be carnivores. That was a lie the meat industry told. He'd seen his dog eat grass: therefore, dogs could live on grass.

No one objected. In fact, others chimed in. My cat eats grass, too, one woman added, all enthusiasm. So does mine! someone else posted. Everyone agreed that fencing was the solution to animal death.

Note well that the site for this liberatory project was Africa. No one mentioned the North American prairie, where carnivores and ruminants alike have been extirpated for the annual grains that vegetarians embrace. But I'll return to that in Chapter 3.

I knew enough to know that this was insane. But no one else on the message board could see anything wrong with the scheme. So, on the theory that many readers lack the knowledge to judge this plan, I'm going to walk you through this.

Carnivores cannot survive on cellulose. They may on occasion eat grass, but they use it medicinally, usually as a purgative to clear their digestive tracts of parasites. Ruminants, on the other hand, have evolved to eat grass. They have a rumen (hence, *ruminant*), the first in a series of multiple stomachs that acts as a fermentative vat. What's actually happening inside a cow or a wildebeest is that bacteria eat the grass, and the animals eat the bacteria.

Lions and hyenas and humans don't have a ruminant's digestive system. Literally from our teeth to our rectums we are designed for meat.[8] We have no mechanism to digest cellulose.

So on the carnivore side of the fence, starvation will take every animal. Some will last longer than others, and those some will end their days as cannibals. The scavengers will have a Fat Tuesday party, but when the bones are picked clean, they'll starve as well. The graveyard won't end there. Without grazers to eat the grass, the land will eventually turn to desert.

Why? Because without grazers to literally level the playing field, the perennial plants mature, and shade out the basal growth point at the plant's base. In a brittle environment like the Serengeti, decay is mostly physical (weathering) and chemical (oxidative), not bacterial and biological as in a moist environment. In fact, the ruminants take over most of the biological functions of soil by digesting the cellulose and returning the nutrients, once again available, in the form of urine and feces.

But without ruminants, the plant matter will pile up, reducing growth, and begin killing the plants. The bare earth is now exposed to wind, sun, and rain, the minerals leach away, and the soil structure is destroyed. In our attempt to save animals, we've killed everything.

On the ruminant side of the fence, the wildebeests and friends will reproduce as effectively as ever. But without the check of predators, there will quickly be more grazers than grass. The animals will outstrip their food source, eat the plants down to the ground, and then starve to death, leaving behind a seriously degraded landscape.

The lesson here is obvious, though it is profound enough to inspire a religion: we need to be eaten as much as we need to eat. The grazers need their daily cellulose, but the grass also needs the animals. It needs the manure, with its nitrogen, minerals, and bacteria; it needs the mechanical check of grazing activity; and it needs the resources stored in animal bodies and freed up by degraders when animals die.

The grass and the grazers need each other as much as predators and prey. These are not one-way relationships, not arrangements of dominance and subordination. We aren't exploiting each other by eating. We are only taking turns.

That was my last visit to the vegan message boards. I realized then that people so deeply ignorant of the nature of life, with its mineral cycle and carbon trade, its balance points around an ancient circle of producers, consumers, and degraders, weren't going to be able to guide me or, indeed, make any useful decisions about sustainable human culture. By turning from adult knowledge, the knowledge that death is embedded in every creature's sustenance, from bacteria to grizzly bears, they would never be able to feed the emotional and spiritual hunger that ached in me from accepting that knowledge. Maybe in the end this book is an attempt to soothe that ache myself.

I have other reasons for writing this book. One is boredom. I'm tired of having the same discussion, especially when it's not an easy discussion to have. Vegetarians can sum up their program in neat sound bites—Meat Is Murder—and self-evident solutions, like those compelling sixteen pounds of grain. I could come up with my own slogans—Monocrops Are Murder? The Million Microbe March?—but they aren't understandable to the general public. I have to start from the beginning, from the first proteins self-organizing into life, moving to photosynthesis, plants, animals, bacteria, soil, and finally agriculture. I call this chat "Microbes, Manure, and Monocrops," and I need a good thirty minutes for the backstory, which is essentially a basic education in the nature of life. And yes, this is information—material, emotional, spiritual—we all should have been given by the time we were four. But who is there left to teach us? And isn't everything that's wrong with this culture embedded in that question?

But it's not just the amount of information that makes the discussion hard. Often, the listener doesn't want to hear it, and the resistance can be extreme. "Vegetarian" isn't just what you eat or even what you believe. It's *who you are*, and it's a totalizing identity. In presenting a fuller picture of food politics, I'm not just questioning a philosophy or a set of dietary habits. I'm threatening a vegetarian's sense of self. And most of you will react with defensiveness and anger. I got hate mail before I'd barely started this book. And no, thank you, I don't need any more.

But I'm also writing this book as a cautionary tale. A vegetarian diet—especially a low-fat version, and most especially a vegan one—is not sufficient nutrition for long-term maintenance and repair of the human body. To put it bluntly, it will damage you. I know. Two years into my veganhood, my health failed, and it failed catastrophically. I developed a degenerative joint disease that I will have for the rest of my life. It started that spring as a strange, dull ache deep in a place I didn't know could have sensation. By the end of the summer, it felt like shrapnel in my spine.

There followed years of ever increasing pain and ever more frustrating visits to specialists. It took fifteen years to get a diagnosis instead of a pat on the head. Teenagers' spines don't fall apart for no reason and so, despite my perfect symptom description, none of the doctors considered Degenerative Disc Disease. Now I've got pictures, and I get respect. My spine looks like a sky-diving accident. Nutritionally, that's about what happened.

Six weeks into veganism I had my first experience of hypoglycemia, though I wouldn't know that's what it was called until eighteen years had gone by and it had become my life. Three months into it I stopped menstruating, which should have been a clue that maybe this wasn't such a good idea. The exhaustion began around then, too, and it only got worse, along with the ever-present cold. My skin was so dry it flaked, and in the winter it itched so badly it kept me up at night. At twenty-four, I developed gastroparesis, which, again, wasn't diagnosed or treated until I was thirty-eight and found a doctor who worked with recovering vegans. That was fourteen years of constant nausea, and I still can't eat after 5 PM.

Then there was the depression and anxiety. I come from a long and venerable line of depressive alcoholics, so clearly I didn't inherit the best mental health genetics. Malnutrition was the last thing I needed. Veganism wasn't the only cause of my depression, but it was a big contributing factor. Years went by when the world was made of a pointless, grey weight, endlessly the same, punctuated only by occasional panic. I would routinely dissolve into helplessness. If I couldn't find my house keys, I'd find myself in a heap on the living room floor, immobilized on the edge of The Void. How could I go on? Why would I want to? The keys were lost and so was I, the world, the cosmos. Everything collapsed, empty, meaningless, almost repulsive. I knew it wasn't rational, but I couldn't stop until it had run its course. And now I know why. Serotonin is made from the amino acid tryptophan. And there are no good plant sources of tryptophan. On top of that, all the tryptophan in the world won't do you any good without saturated fat, which is necessary to make your neurotransmitters actually transmit. All those years of emotional collapse weren't a personal failing; they were bio-chemical, if self-inflicted.

Is there anything as boring as other people's medical problems? I'll try to keep this brief. My spine isn't coming back. But eating a diet of grass-fed animal products has repaired the damage a bit and made a moderate dent in my pain level. My insulin receptors are also down for the count, but protein and fat keep my blood sugar stable and happy. I haven't missed a period in five years, though if I end up with cancer in my reproductive organs, I'm blaming soy. My stomach's okay—not great, but okay—as long as I take betaine hydrochloride with every meal. Between my spiritual practice and my nutrient-dense diet, I am now depression-free, and I am thankful every day. But the cold and the exhaustion are permanent. Some days breathing takes more energy than I have.

You don't have to try this for yourself. You're allowed to learn from my mistakes. All the friends of my youth were radical, righteous, intense. Vegetarianism was the obvious path, with veganism the high road alongside it. And those of us who did it long term ended up damaged. If I'm questioning your lifestyle, your identity, you might feel confusion, fear, and anger while reading this book. But take my word: you don't want to end up like me. I'm asking you to stay the course, read this book, and explore the resources in the appendix. Please. Especially if you have children or want to. I'm not too proud to beg.

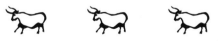

Smokers will tell you that there is nothing like an ex-smoker. The urge to proselytize the Good News seems to flow with the attainment of salvation, or maybe in their case, with oxygen. I have done my best to avoid a tone of moral superiority and aim for engagement. I hope I have succeeded. Ultimately I would rather be helpful than right. Especially considering the future we are facing and how much is at stake. The underlying values that vegetarians claim to honor—justice, compassion, sustainability—are the only values that will create a world of connection instead of domination; a world where humans approach every creature—every rock, every raindrop, all our furred and feathered siblings—with humility, awe, and respect; the only world with a chance of surviving the abuse called civilization. It is in the hope that such a world is possible that I offer this book.

CHAPTER 2
Moral Vegetarians

Start with an apple. A food so nonviolent it wants to be eaten, say the fruitarians, people who try to live by fruit alone, or die in the attempt. Some plants surround their seeds with pulpy sweetness wrapped in bright colors to tempt animals to eat them, and, in the eating, to carry the seeds to new, potentially fertile, ground. Animals do the work that plants can't do, rooted as they are to one spot: find a possible place for their young to grow.

So eating an apple is okay to these most moral of vegetarians, since no death is involved. Or so the story goes.

The first problem is that humans don't plant those seeds. We discard them. We consciously remove the core to avoid the seeds and then throw them away—"away" in industrial nations meaning sealed in a plastic bag that gets entombed in a landfill. Or factories squeeze or chop the fruit for us, rendering it into juice or McPies, dumping the peels and pulp and seeds nowhere near a nice pile of manure in a clearing.[1]

Or, if we're extra eco-righteous, we throw the seeds on the compost heap, where time, heat and bacteria kill them. One goal of any good compost scheme, after all, is to kill any lingering seeds.

None of this is what the tree had in mind.

The tree isn't offering sweetness out of the goodness of its heartwood. It's striking a bargain, and even though we've shaken hands and collected, we aren't carrying through on our side of the deal.

There's a glaring anthropocentrism in this argument, which is strange coming from people espousing a specific politic of animal liberation. "The fruit tree gives me my food and I give back the seeds to nature so other trees can grow," writes one vegetarian.[2] Yes, but he isn't giving the seeds back to nature. Why are we humans allowed to take without giving? Isn't that called exploitation? Or at the very least, stealing? Fruit isn't, as claimed, "the only freely given food."[3] The point of that fruit is not humans. The point is the seeds. The reason that the tree expends such tremendous resources accumulating fibers and sugars is to secure the best possible future for its offspring. And we take that offspring, in its swaddling of sweetness, and kill it.

This is not what vegetarians want to hear, at least not the ones I'm calling moral vegetarians. There are other branches of the vegetarian tree—political vegetarians who believe a plant-based diet is more just and sustainable, and nutritional vegetarians who believe that animal products are the root of all dietary evil—and I'll be addressing those arguments in later chapters. But the moral argument is the clarion call that rallies most vegetarians to the cause. It's what kept me unable to examine or even question my vegan diet, despite all evidence that my health was failing. I wanted to believe that my life—my physical existence—was possible without killing, without death. It's not. No life is. But since fairy tales are filled with apples, let's continue to follow their crumbs through the fruit-filled forest.

These lead right to the second problem: there are no apples in nature. Apples are domesticated. Apples started as *Malus sieversii*, in the mountains of Kazakhstan and, once upon a time, they were bitter.

"Imagine sinking your teeth into a tart potato or a slightly mushy Brazil nut covered in leather," writes Michael Pollan of tasting true wild apples. "On the first bite some of these apples would start out with high promise on the tongue—*Now here's an apple!*—only to suddenly veer into a bitterness so profound it makes my stomach rise even at the recollection."[4]

This is true of most domestic fruits. Their progenitors are almost inedible by humans.

"The fruit tree gives me my food and I give back the seeds to nature so other trees can grow."[5] Really? Dare you. Because most trees that produce edible fruit—and definitely apples—don't come from seeds. If you actually were to plant the seeds, most of the wildlings that sprouted would be unpalatable to humans. Fruit trees are grafted, not sprouted.[6]

The "natural" food of humans doesn't exist in nature. If we are now lost (and starving) in the inedible forest, maybe it's because our moral map was wrong.

To say there is a "freely given food" implies there is a giver—the tree, the cane, the stalk of wheat. To believe in food that requires "No killing or theft from animal or plant"[7] is to recognize that plants and animals love their lives, and their body parts, whether fibrous or muscular. But not their offspring? The argument fails right here. If we believe in their sentience, why not in the sentience of their babies? If it's wrong to steal from a plant, why isn't it more wrong to kill a seed? We can't have it both ways. Either there is a giver, a being deserving our reciprocity, or there isn't. If killing is the problem, the life of one grass-fed cow will feed me for an entire year. But a single vegan meal of plant babies—rice grains, almonds, soybeans—ground up or boiled alive, will involve hundreds of deaths. Why don't they matter?

"I won't eat anything that has a mother or a face," was one of my standard declarations. But every living thing has a mother. Some of them have fathers, too. Why didn't I know that? What I meant was: I won't eat anything that was nurtured by its mother, which meant, essentially, birds and mammals, though I didn't eat seafood either. Some beings give their lives to produce their offspring. That means they can't be around to nurture them, but does that mean they love their offspring any less? Motherhood—and sometimes fatherhood—as the ultimate sacrifice. Wouldn't that action imply they loved their offspring the most? And suppose your mother didn't love you: does that mean your life is intrinsically worth less?

Then there's the face part. Why does the possession of a face define who counts or who doesn't? What it actually defines is who is most like humans, who more different: do they look like us? There's that anthropocentrism again, an ethical system based on how similar a living being is to humans. Why is that what matters? Why are humans the standard that measures who lives and who dies?

An apple falls from the tree. We eat its sweetness and, despite dis-ingenuous claims to the contrary, kill the seeds. One could argue that in an earlier age, humans acted as unwitting cultivators, seed-bearers, spitting or shitting out the bitter pits, some of which would take root. We weren't always stealing and killing apple offspring. Perhaps if the asphalt was removed and the earth restored, the underlying reciproc-ity of the human-apple relationship would naturally reassert itself.

But humans can't live on apples. And in the vegetarian moral universe, all seeds—nuts, grains—are seen as freely given. In the case of these seeds, there is no tasty pulp in exchange for baby-on-board. It's *the seeds themselves* that humans eat. I remember my reasoning: annual grasses died anyway at harvest time, so I wasn't *really* killing. The problem, of course, is that I wasn't eating the part that died: the stalk. Humans can't digest cellulose. I was eating the precise part that wants very much to live: the seed. In fact, they want to live so much that even after thousands of dormant years, some of them will sprout. Who can say this is a being who doesn't love its life?

I know from experience that the issue of plants and their sen-tience is thrown at vegetarians by detractors all the time. I know how smug and hostile those detractors usually are. The idea of respecting plants is just as ridiculous to them as the idea of respecting animals. They argue as devil's advocates. But I am not advocating for any devil. He clearly can do his own work just fine. I mean to address these concerns seriously. I hear a plea in the words of vegetarians, a plea that borders on a prayer. *Let me live without harm to others. Let my life be possible without death.* This prayer embodies both a fierce tender-ness and a passionate repugnance. The love is for all beings, and the horror is for the sadism humans are inflicting. This prayer pulses in me like another heart. What separates me from vegetarians isn't ethics or commitment. It's information.

Because I have grown apples and I know what goes into them. I can go to the local feed store and buy a bag of Organic Fertilizer for Fruit Trees and ask no more. But it's not in my nature to skip the fine print. I want to know. I read the labels. My passion to live a good life, an honorable and ethical life, had propelled me to start growing as much of my own food as possible. I knew that the three most important ecological actions that we can take as individuals are: refrain from having children, don't drive a car, grow your own food. I wasn't in contact with the leading cause of pregnancy; I was too poor to own a car; that left growing my food.

I didn't attempt my first garden under duress. The idea of gardening entered my mind like a sliver of sunrise. If you have had depression, then you know how anything that makes you feel something is a miracle. Where the world was a flat, chronic grey, the garden brought life. And it overflowed with green. I wrapped small seeds in moist cloth and two days later a tiny finger, as tentative as hope, reached from each one. They wanted to live and so did I. I spent long New England nights under a heavy weight of covers, rallying against the physical pain that never ended, only ebbed, and the depression that, like the cold, was everywhere and always hungry. All that protruded into the hostile air was my head and one hand, holding a seed catalog like a white flag signaling for mercy. And the garden did bring mercy. Things grew, climbed, bloomed, fruited, an inexorable and silent song of green, an endless circle of yearning that was so much bigger than me, my pain. I found solace in the garden and tiny moments of joy that appeared suddenly, wondrously, like the violets and bachelor's buttons that volunteered every spring without any help from me.

I discovered *Organic Gardening* magazine and, even better, that the library would let me check out the back issues. I read them all. I filled a notebook with my small, earnest print. I was so innocent. Had I really not known that tomatoes couldn't go out until after frost? Memorial Day, I wrote, then underlined. Did I really not know that beans couldn't be transplanted, that snapdragons were annuals?

With my spine, there could be no digging, no lifting, not much physical labor at all. But that was okay. I immediately searched out the garden techniques that were the most radical, the most sustainable. Ruth Stout was a revelation.[8] So was permaculture.[9] I would use wide beds, permanent mulch. I would build topsoil from the top down, like nature. There would be no tilling, no bare soil, no double digging. The realization that the rationale behind these techniques was really an indictment of annual grains—of agriculture itself—I left for another day.

There were other things I didn't know, even more basic than planting zones and growing seasons. There was knowledge that I sought, but then refused: I wasn't the only one eating. The plants were hungry, too. And then there was the soil. Feed the soil, the garden books urged. Was the soil actually eating? What was soil? Was it, too, alive?

One tablespoon of soil contains more than one million living organisms, and, yes, every one of them is eating. Soil isn't just dirt. A square meter of topsoil can contain a thousand different *species* of animals.[10] These might include 120 million nematodes, 100,000 mites, 45,000 springtails, 20,000 enchytraeid worms, and 10,000 molluscs.[11]

All those tiny creatures live in and around humus, which is a combination of humic acid and polysaccharides. "No one knows how humic acid forms, but once formed it acts like a living substance," writes Stephen Harrod Buhner.[12] More life. How far down did I have to dig to stop finding living creatures? Because if it was alive, I couldn't kill it. I read that "[v]ery small animals are able to live a basically aquatic life in soil, in the water found attached to soil crumbs."[13] There was a whole world under my feet, a world that included its own ocean. A world where the real work of life—producing and degrading—was being done. Animals like me were just consumers, hitching along for the ride. I couldn't photosynthesize—turn sun into mass—nor could I turn that mass back into carbon and minerals. They could and they did, and because of them, life was possible. I was made humble.

But I had bet my whole moral system—and built my whole identity—on the idea that my life did not require death. The more I learned, the more questions I had to ignore if I wanted to save this ethical directive that claimed to be about facing the truth. Did the lives of nematodes and fungi matter? Why not? Because they were too small for me to see? Because they were on the other side of an intellectual Maginot Line of us/them? But I was supposed to be one of the brave ones who refused to draw that line, who didn't put humans above animals in a hierarchy, who reverenced the natural world and all capital-H Her creatures.

But this only included the creatures that were like me in certain, very specific ways. I saw that in tiny flashes, each new piece of information flickering like a firefly. Those instants of light signaled a dark forest that I refused to enter. I kept turning instead toward what I knew, a rosary of statistics that was my penance and protection. The pounds of grain, the gallons of water, the hungry bellies. I was on the side of righteousness, and like any fundamentalist, I could only stay there by avoiding information.

So humic acid—creature of mystery, very much alive—breaks down plant compounds and stores them inside itself. When it gets the right signals from its ecosystem it recombines and releases the needed nutrients. "Through tightly coupled feedback processes information on the chemistry reserves stored in humic acid feeds back into the above ground plant communities, indicating what plants should grow in what combination in what ecosystem and what kind of chemistries they should produce to keep the soil healthy."[14]

The soil wasn't a thing, it was a million things, and they were alive. Their life processes—eating, excreting, tunneling, communicating, exchanging—were what made the rest of the planet livable. They broke down dead matter from plants, animals, fungi, bacteria and made the constituent elements available for more life. Steven Stoll writes that topsoil "is a filter and a container, a mass of integrated micro and macro matter, and a living substance that cannot be understood by reduction. Its final form contains so many members and symbiotic relationships that it constitutes, in the words of the soil scientist Nyle Brady, the 'genesis of a natural body distinct from the parent materials from which the body was formed.'"[15]

"Feed the soil, not the plant," was the first commandment of organic growing. I had to feed the soil because it was alive.

Nitrogen, phosphorus, potassium—NPK—is the Triple Goddess of gardeners, the Troika of elements that rule plant growth. What did soil and plants eat and where would I get those substances? I hadn't learned the phrase "closed-loop system," but that was what I was after. Nitrogen was the big one. There are plants that fix nitrogen. Wasn't that enough for my garden? Couldn't it be? I begged. But I was begging a million living creatures who had organized themselves into

mutual dependence millions of years ago. They had no use for my
ethical anguish. No nitrogen-fixing plant could make up for all the
nutrients I was taking out. The soil wanted manure. Worse, it wanted
the inconceivable: blood and bones.

There were other sources of nitrogen I could have applied. Right
now, fossil fuel provides the nitrogen to grow crops the world over.
Synthetic fertilizer is what created the green revolution, with its 250
percent increase in crops. Besides the fact that nothing made from
fossil fuels is sustainable—we can't grow fossil fuel and it doesn't reproduce itself—synthetic fertilizers eventually destroy the soil.

So synthetic nitrogen was out. And that left me facing animal
products. Of course, the irony is that either source of nitrogen, synthetic or organic, comes from animals. Oil and gas are what's left of
the dinosaurs. So my choices—our choices, actually—were nitrogen
from dead reptiles or from living ruminants.

My garden wanted to eat animals, even if I didn't.

So I came to another fork in my Pilgrimage Road. I could buy
a box of condensed NPK, nicely balanced and all organic, or I could
make friends with a dairy farmer. The box was tempting, because I
could lie. No, not quite lie. I could not-know what I already knew. I
could refuse the information. Because I already knew what was in that
box. The list of ingredients glimmered and promised like the fruit of
knowledge always does. I was Eve, and here was my apple, and what
would be the cost of eating? The literal cost I had finally come up
against, the bottom line of the mineral cycle? The emotional cost to
my spiritual longings, my political passions, my identity? And why is
it always about eating?

I took a bite. I read the label. Blood meal, bone meal, dead animals, dried and ground. I put the box down and found some manure.
Friends of a friend, a barn now empty of goats but filled with manure.
It turned out I knew the woman who had owned the goats and she
was a decent person. Her animals would have been well cared for, in-
dulged even. I was dating someone with a pickup truck and a strong
back. The manure arrived and my garden exploded. The tomato vines
swallowed their trellises, then their bed, then developed designs on
the driveway. It looked like the Land That Time Forgot outside my

back window. I fed three households on the produce and still, some of the lettuce bolted before we got to it.[16]

And I was left hungry as well as nourished. This was not an anticipatory hunger, the smell of dinner at the front door, a lover's look of longing across a crowded room. This was a hunger that gnawed with no promise of relief. I was closing the loop in my garden now, but my ethical system had broken open.

Years later, I would have a discussion with an earnest young vegan.

"They take dead chicken parts and spread them on the fields." His voice was shaking. He assumed I'd sympathize, that anyone with my politics would automatically be appalled. His eco-pure, non-violent, plant-based diet was being violated by the forces of evil, of death.

"Plants have to eat, too," I tried to explain. "They need nitrogen, they need minerals. You have to replace what you're taking out. Your choices are fossil fuels or animal products."

"But—but—" Now his body was trembling as well as his voice. I knew what he wanted to say. *It's not true. It can't be true. There's a way out of death and I've found it.*

"No," was the only word he could come up with. Then he walked away.

How many times did I walk away? Over and over and over. But I couldn't walk away from my garden, from my attempts to not be a parasite on the planet. So while I closed the nutrient cycle, I had nowhere to go with the information I was using for that task. I could play intellectual hide and seek over the goat manure—it was already there, piled in the barn, why not use it, *I* wasn't the one oppressing animals for milk and meat—but the P and K in NPK weren't so easily avoided.

Globally, phosphorus is available in extremely limited quantities. "Next to clean water," writes Bill Mollison, "phosphorus will be one of the inexorable limits to human occupancy on this planet."[17] It exists in sedimentary rock. I didn't put rocks in the same category as animals: I didn't mind using them. The problem was getting them. They had to be quarried—mined—then ground up, and transported.

Without vast amounts of fossil fuels, would that even be possible? And what about when we'd used it all up? I was back to the same shelf at the feed store. I could buy rock phosphate, decide that because it was "organic" I was doing the good, green thing and simply not think about it anymore. But wasn't there a sustainable source I could get on my own? I asked the question, but hated the answer.

"Bone meal from land animals is a traditional source, and most farms (up to 1940) kept a flock of pigeons as their source." Or I could theoretically get it from "seabirds and salmon [who] do try to recycle it back to us but we tend to reduce their numbers by denying them breeding grounds."[18] I was ninety miles from the ocean. I was barely a mile from the Connecticut River, one of the southernmost habitats for Atlantic salmon, but there haven't been anadramous fish in the Connecticut since the river was dammed almost two hundred years ago, to power the mills.

And then there was K, potassium, available in ash, bones, urine, manure and some cover crops. I could pretend I'd find a supply of ash— woodstoves being as ubiquitous as maple trees in western Massachusetts— and grow some cover crops, but I think by the time I got to K I was too intellectually exhausted to bother. My food had to eat before I ate it.

There were finer points, all of them sharp and hungry, that I learned about growing fruit. I didn't have fruit trees yet, but they were part of the mythic farm that waited in my mist-shrouded future. Calcium is always a limiting factor in the soil. When the calcium is gone, growth stops. And again, the calcium would come from ... Would I finish the sentence with an organic box from the feed store, laden with embodied energy and slaughterhouse dust? Or would I learn the grammar of my great-grandparents, and feed the trees with the bones of animals that lived beside me? Would there be any solace in this information? I found one small comfort in *The Apple Grower* by Michael Phillips. He quotes a book called *The Apple Culturist* from 1871, recounting the story of an apple tree near the graves of Roger Williams, the founder of Rhode Island, and his wife Mary Sayles. The roots of the tree were found to have grown into the graves and assumed the shape of human skeletons while "the graves [were] emptied of every particle of human dust. Not a trace of anything was left."[19]

This story eased my mind, because the tree ate the humans. The standard narrative of Man the Hunter was repugnant to me, with its biological determinism, its celebration of dominance, violence, rape, death. The myth always ends with Man on top: of animals, women, the food chain, the planet. It may be a political reality, but there's a name for it—patriarchy—and a solution—organized resistance. I rejected the assertion that hierarchy was inevitable, that the Cosmos had chosen humans as the pinnacle, that men had to be men. And I like to believe I'd have rejected this propaganda just as firmly if I were a man, though I know that the privileges of power make that less likely.

Even the people who should know better fall for the Man as Apex myth. At a groovy Earth Day gathering, a line of costumed dancers was supposed to represent the food chain, starting with plants and ending with humans. But it doesn't end with us, I kept insisting to anyone who'd listen, mostly my companions who got tired of hearing it. What about the scavengers, the coyotes, the carrion birds? What about the insects, the maggots, the bacteria? We're not at the end because it's not a line. It's a circle, and if it ends anywhere it's with the degraders feeding the producers. We're just a juicy snack.

But I couldn't listen to that apple tree, speaking in slow, slow sign with its skeleton roots, saying: you are the exact shape of my hunger. Our animal bones, our human blood; we belong here too, if we're willing to accept our place. We are eaten as well as eaters, raw materials for the endless feast. That would have been the solace: a place at the table. We aren't above, just one among many beings embraced by carbon that one day will let go.

But I had to accept death before I could take my place.

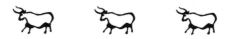

I wish I could go back ten years and tell my younger self: the day will come when you have a flock of pigeons, and you'll spread their manure and bury their dead among the berries and apples. And you'll cry when you do it, but not just because it's sad. Because it's holy and it's been done well. You've closed the circle, and it will open your heart. You'll have chickens, too, and ducks, geese, guineas. They'll eat the bugs. You'll eat the fruit, the eggs, the meat. They'll accept you—come to you for help and for cuddle sessions—and you'll love them. And you'll eat, all of you, birds, berries, humans, soil, and be eaten. Since sky burials are illegal, it'll be in your will: scatter my ashes when it's my turn, feed the berries and the apples.

Would it have helped to hear that, or would the horror at what I would become—eater of meat, murderer—leave no room for blaze marks on the long, heavy path to grace? I want to tell myself: you will eat strawberries so full each one is an epiphany, every bite a communion, well beyond forgiveness and redemption. Each taste will bring you home. That is the only fruit worth eating, tart as well as sweet, plump with life that grows from death, that blooms and ripens in its season.

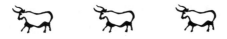

Which brings us back to apples. *The fruit tree gives me my food and I give back the seeds to nature so other trees can grow.* The last time I ate an apple, I counted. There were ten seeds. Set aside for a moment that those seeds won't produce edible apples: even if the fruitarian has a really big backyard, he would have run out of space long ago. He didn't mean it literally. He couldn't. But I keep coming back to this sentence because there is something in it that matters to the author, and it's the thing that matters to me: relationship, and one of mutuality and respect. The author clearly yearns for food—for a life—based on reciprocity, not exploitation, and he believes that plants count as partners, as participants. Having included them in the "us" of sentience and agency, he can't just take. He needs to know that he is giving back, part of a circle of exchange, instead of the one-way extraction that he identifies as death. This sentence embodies one of the impulses that is salutary in the vegetarian myth: the attempt to take humans down from our destructive perch as lords above and return us to our honest place in a circle.

But it also reflects the ignorance. He doesn't know that apples eat, and what they eat is animals, including us. They need our excrement—the nitrogen, the minerals, the microbes—and our flesh and bones. There is a reciprocal relationship between animals and plants: predator and prey, until the prey becomes predator. It is only our attempt to remove ourselves from that cycle that destroys it.

There's more ignorance. He doesn't know that seeds are alive. Or he won't let himself. Since killing is the sacrilege in this moral system, he can't acknowledge that in actuality he's eating something alive. This, despite the fact that he sees plants as beings deserving his respect.

And there is a final ignorance in his misapprehension of the nature of apple trees. There is a relationship of reciprocity built into the human-apple exchange, but it's not about humans planting their seeds. It's about humans grafting, planting, and tending the trees and extending their territory. It's about apples tempting us, with an offer of sweetness, to toil for them. It's a coevolutionary process, and it's called domestication.

Domestication is not a concept that's well understood by people who claim to be against it. I saw domestication as bringing animals and plants under human control and it was appalling to me, a short trajectory that ended in hens tormented in battery cages and primates brutalized in head injury experiments. Of course, my entire diet was composed of domesticates, with the exception of a serving or two of fiddlehead ferns every spring, but they were plants, so I simply didn't think about it. It was the animals I wanted to save from human exploitation, and in the vegan outlook, exploitation begins with domestication.

There was an exact moment when that definition cracked open for me. It was six o'clock on a January morning, and well below zero. I had a half gallon of hot water to haul through three feet of ice-slick snow so that my chickens would have something to drink. Water had dripped into the doorjamb the warm day before and then frozen the door shut in the night. Never mind the long task involving screwdrivers, butter knives, and matches to unthaw the door. Somewhere between burning my palm and feeling a hideous blob of snow hit the back of my neck, I thought: I've had it backward all these years. I'm not exploiting them. They're happy, safe, warm, and fed. I'm the one who's miserable. Chickens won't even walk in snow, let alone haul supplies to me. That wet drip sliding down my spine was like a cold jab of reality. Chickens have gotten humans to work for them. In exchange, they take care of us, but not by bringing us water. By providing food—meat and eggs—and a whole constellation of other activities useful for farms. It's a partnership, and one that worked out well for both parties until factory-farming. The genome of the jungle fowl took a chance on humans and it was a gamble that paid off. We have carried chickens all over the globe, extending their range beyond the wildest dreams of a broody jungle fowl mom, ready and willing to give all to her eggs.

This is the main point of Michael Pollan's marvelous book, *The Botany of Desire: A Plant's-Eye View of the World.*

> We automatically think of domestication as something we do to other species, but it makes just as much sense to think of it as something that certain plants and animals have done to us, a clever evolutionary strategy for advancing their own interests. The species that have spent the last ten thousand or so years figuring out how best to feed, heal, clothe, intoxicate, and otherwise delight us have made themselves some of nature's greatest success stories.[20]

An example? He points to the US's fifty million dogs versus ten thousand wolves.[21] Wild canines found a better life beside humans. To begin with, there was a lot of meat to scavenge. And the more canines helped humans, the more they tracked and chased and took down prey with us, the more food there was.

There are two million named species of animals on the planet, and countless more awaiting identification. Only *forty* have linked their futures to ours. We changed them—asked them to be bigger, smaller, faster, gentler—and they changed us. Half of all humans now possess the lactose tolerance gene, the biological result of the bovine experiment on humans. And our whole way of life changed, from hunter-gatherers to horticulturalists and sedentary agriculturalists. All because we liked something that certain animals and plants offered us.

Of 422,000 plant species, only a tiny percentage are domesticates. But some of those have literally taken over the globe. Plants
produce millions of chemicals to attract, repel, immobilize, or kill
animals. It's how some of them reproduce. And it's how they fight
back: nature, red in phytochemicals. Just because they can't locomote
doesn't mean they're passive. And every so often in the evolutionary
crapshoot, one of them throws the gene dice and beats the house,
producing a perfect match with the pleasure centers in the human
brain. Annual grasses hit pay dirt with their opioids. We ate them and
couldn't stop. "Our grammar," writes Michael Pollan, "might teach
us to divide the world into active subjects and passive objects, but
in a coevolutionary relationship every subject is also an object, every
object a subject. That's why it makes just as much sense to think of
agriculture as something the grasses did to people as a way to conquer
the trees."[22]

We supplied the brute force. As far as corn is concerned, we're
just the draft horses.

We need to take ourselves out of the subject position. We need
to realize that we aren't so special. We think we do this human-only
activity—changing plants and animals to suit our needs until they're
dependent on us. But *all* predators change their prey, and all prey
is dependent on predators. Do you think chameleons switch colors
for fun, that fawns have spots and an instinct to lie perfectly still just
because?

Currently, the deer are overrunning the northeast's forests, eating
the saplings out of existence. In fifty years there may not be a forest,
and that will mean an end to the deer as well. That's because, through
human interference, there aren't enough predators, and to survive, the
deer need their predators. Pollan explains, "[H]owever it may appear
to those of us living at such a remove from the natural world, predation is not a matter of morality or of politics; it, too, is a matter of
symbiosis ... Predation is deeply woven into the fabric of nature, and

that fabric would quickly unravel if it somehow ended, if humans managed to 'do something about it.'"[23] In the case of the northeastern United States, humans *have* managed to do something about it, and without wolves and mountain lions, without predation, the results are getting grimmer by the year. The deer population has exploded past any possibility of sustainability. Writes Ted Williams:

> In a 10-year experiment, the US Forest Service found that at more than 20 deer per square mile you lose your eastern wood pewees, indigo buntings, least flycatchers, yellow-billed cuckoos, and cerulean warblers .... At 38 deer per square mile you lose eastern phoebes and even robins. Ground nesters like ovenbirds, grouse, woodcock, whippoorwills, and wild turkeys can nest in ferns, which deer scorn, but these birds, too, are vastly reduced, because they need thick cover.[24]

He describes Crane Estate, a barrier-beach north of Boston, completely stripped of native plants, its bare dunes lost to the wind, and the rest of the wildlife along with them. The deer themselves were starving, having long overshot the land's carrying capacity, and were in the process of permanently degrading it. Without predators, the land dies. In this case, those predators, mainly cougars and wolves, were killed off by the early European settlers. "This behavior flabbergasted the Indians," writes Williams. "After much arguing and theorizing, they decided it was a symptom of insanity."

Predator-prey is ultimately a mutual relationship: each needs the other, changes the other. Writes Pollan, "Human hunting ... literally helped form the American Plains bison, which ... changed both physically and behaviorally after the arrival of the Indians."[25] *And large ruminants changed humans just as surely as we changed them.* The high-quality proteins and fats, especially the nutrient-dense organ meats, meant our digestive systems could shrink and our brains could grow. The megafauna of the prehistoric world, the aurochs and antelopes and mammoths, literally made us human. There is a reason they were our first, endless art project.

As for plants, they've been using animals as a reproductive strategy for 100 million years, since the angiosperms literally blossomed on the evolutionary scene. Some plants now reproduce by creating flowers. These flowers need animals to pollinate them. Once fertilized, the flowers turn into seeds, seeds that in turn need animals to carry them. Some plants harnessed the wind as pollinator and as transport, and the tiny fairy parachutes of milk thistle are the results. Others learned to attract animals; sex, from the beginning, has been an orgy of color and scent and taste, brilliant red for hummingbirds, sweet nectar for bees. These plants coevolved with their animal cohorts. They are as dependent on insects, birds, and rodents as corn is on humans. For instance:

> Several species of acacia trees, known as ant acacias, have a highly developed relationship with certain ant species. In the case of Acacia cornigera and the ant Pseudomyrmex ferruginea, each species depends absolutely on its relationship with the other.... The tree has swollen thorns in which the ants hollow out nests. Its leaf stalks produce a nectar that provides the ants with carbohydrates they need; special bright orange growths at the tips of the leaflets ... supply the ants with protein and fat.... The queen of an acacia ant colony finds an unoccupied acacia seedling and burrows into a green thorn, where she lays her eggs .... Within nine months of the queen's arrival, the workers are patrolling the tree, walking up and down the branches and leaves day and night. They attack— biting and stinging—any other insects they find, and they kill any plants that grow within a thirty-inch radius of their tree.... Young ant acacias that do not have an ant colony suffer severe damage from other insects.... In fact ant acacias depend on 'their' ants for survival.[26]

Domestication is not human domination. Yes, now we understand the mechanics of genes and breeding, and we like to believe we are in charge. You can insist that humans are on top—in control, self-conscious—but wheat and corn, from their 850-million-acre position around the globe, would argue otherwise. And they've got our back-breaking labor and shrunken skeletons to prove it.

🐂   🐂   🐂

Whether life on earth is one organism, and whether all of it is conscious, are ultimately spiritual questions. I don't think the answers can be argued, only experienced. And I've had my experiences. I know what I believe. I'm not asking you to agree with me, only to observe. Squirrels bury acorns. Oak trees feed squirrels. Monarch butterflies need asclepias, and not just for the sugar. Asclepias produce a specific chemical in their nectar that render monarchs toxic to their predators. Who is working for whom? Human relationships with chickens and pigs, rice and barley, are no different.

The first requirement for domestication is a plant willing to stretch its genome to fit a human need. Humans harvest, unintentionally disburse, and protect the plant. These are activities common to hunter-gatherers, and they result in genetic changes to malleable, agreeable plants, like larger seeds and non-shattering rachises. Such plants become more attractive to, but also more dependent on, humans. David Rindos calls this stage *incidental domestication.*[27] The next stage occurs when plants need humans to disperse them, and humans engage in specific behaviors to encourage the domesticate. Rindos calls this *specialized domestication.* The archaeological record shows corresponding changes in seed size, coatings, and dispersal mechanisms. The landscape also changes due to human activity, although these activities are still in the province of hunter-gatherers (usually burning and clearing). A diversity of wild plant species is still present as the domesticates do not provide enough sustenance and humans are still dependent on other resources. In the final stage, *agricultural domestication*, domesticates out-produce wild plants and humans engage in full-scale altering of environments for the sake of domesticates. At this point, species diversity plunges, and humans are dependent on fully domesticated plants and animals.

In order for full-scale agriculture to occur, three conditions have to be met. First, there must be a suite of appropriate, malleable plants and animals. The available suite is in essence a limiting factor. This is the reason that humans in North America were only able to practice agriculture in small areas. There were no potential megafaunal domesticates. Without domesticable animals, sedentary humans had to rely on rivers, estuaries, and the ocean to provide animal fats and proteins. Outside the river valleys and coastal areas, agriculture wasn't possible. In Meso-America and South America, the llama, as well as the guinea pig and the turkey, were domesticated, and agriculture proceeded in its typical destructive pattern.

Second, the environment has to be rich enough in resources that human population begins to grow. This is important because it leads to the third factor: human disturbance of the environment. As humans gathered in seasonal villages, they would burn the area to set up camp, then trample around a wider area, burn some more to flush out game, and build piles of waste. The domesticable seeds, particularly the annual grasses, were excreted incidentally, spread purposefully, or both, and they were right at home in these disturbed environments. Horticulturalists would plant food-bearing and other useful plants before leaving a site. In the South American rainforest, for instance, over three hundred plants have been domesticated over centuries of this cycle. The rainforest as it exists today is a cooperative effort formed by the interactions of humans and plants.

The key to full-fledged agriculture is the annual grasses. If you want to understand ten thousand years of human-wrought destruction, you have to understand the nature of annual plants. The vast majority of plants on our planet are perennials. Once established, they live for years, sometimes centuries, accumulating sunlight into cellulose. Because they have a lot of time to reproduce, they use multiple strategies: runners, tubers, canes, seeds. Their function in the ecosystem is vital: their roots literally hold the soil in place. And without topsoil, there is no life, or no land life anyway.

Now contrast that to annuals. They only live a short season or two, and in that time they have to complete their life's purpose: reproduction. So they bet the whole farm on one strategy: big, fat seeds. Their seeds are patient because they have to be. There's no point in sprouting when the competition is established perennials. Their tiny little radicles don't stand a chance against a tight mat of perennial roots. They wait until something has destroyed the perennials and bared the soil—fire, flood, earthquake, migrating bison, humans. With the perennial plants temporarily shoved aside, the annuals come into their own. The seeds sprout, roots go down, stalks shoot up, and the plants get to work on getting sexy. They don't have long to send out love letters of shape and color, sweet nothings of pollen and scent, before perennials start closing in and, in temperate climates, winter. So the annuals get themselves fertilized, their seed pods swell and burst, and the next generation of seeds lie waiting in the soil for their disaster. Living proof that nature loves an opportunist.

From the point of view of the soil, nothing could be better. Bare dirt is an emergency and annuals are the first responders, holding and protecting the soil with their bodies of roots and leaves. Annuals are like the band-aid over a wound, while perennials are the flesh that eventually knits back together.

The starting point of agriculture was annual grasses—the wild progenitors of corn, rice, wheat, barley (with the potatoes of the Andes being the tuberous exception)—because they produced seeds big enough to be worth the effort of harvesting. They came into their own in river valleys prone to flooding where they found good niches in the predictable disturbance. Then along came humans, playing with fire, eating and excreting, and the annual grasses were right at home. The plants were camp followers. They liked growing in the disturbed areas humans provided.

Agriculture started in six separate centers with different plants: maize from Central America; rice from the Yellow and Yangtze rivers in China and the Ganges in India; a different species of rice from West Africa; wheat from the Middle East; floodplain weeds (gourds, sunflowers and chenopods) from the south central US; and potatoes from the Andes. All these areas produced agriculture and then, in short order, urban civilizations. This happened not because of human behavior alone, but because of the annual plants that were attracted to human behavior.

That's the how of agriculture. It doesn't explain the why. Why would humans give up a life of near-perfect health and leisure for back-breaking labor and bad nutrition?

The transition to agriculture "has long been celebrated ... as a major advance in civilization, but ... health deteriorated during the changeover."[28] The advent of agriculture leaves almost forensic traces in bones and fecal remnants, evidence of crimes against the basic human template: "malnutrition, osteomyelitis and periostitis (bone infections), intestinal parasites, yaws, syphilis, leprosy, tuberculosis, anemia (from poor diet as well as from hookworms), rickets in children, osteomalacia in adults, retarded childhood growth, and short stature among adults."[29] Medical anthropologists can look at a bone and tell in a glance whether the subject lived in a hunter-gatherer or an agricultural society. The hunters look great. The farmers are falling apart.

And then there's the endless effort. The average hunter-gatherer works seventeen hours a week, which leaves plenty of time for creative endeavors, spiritual concerns, gossiping, and the all-important nap.[30] Agriculturalists work from dawn to dusk and then some, and even in modern America, with all our hallowed technology, the average US citizen works over forty hours a week, which doesn't even include life maintenance tasks (traditionally assigned to women) like cooking, cleaning, and child-rearing. Beastly indeed. Why did humans do it?

Various theories have been put forward, but none of them have stood up to the facts. The one I learned in school was that human population pressure forced people to make their territories more productive. It would make sense if only it were true. If overpopulation were the stressor, then archaeologists would find the brittle, shrunken, and degenerated skeletons of the malnourished *before* evidence of agriculture, but they don't. They find instead the long, strong, disease-free bones and teeth typical of hunter-gatherers. It's after agriculture that human populations swelled past carrying capacity. "Population pressure seems to have played no direct role in early stages of domestication," conclude Douglas T. Price and Anne Birgitte Gebauer.[31]

The archaeologists need to talk to the pharmacologists. Bighorn sheep will chew their teeth down to the gums to eat psychoactive lichen off of rocks. Cattle will return to eat locoweed until it kills them. Birds get stoned on cannabis seeds, and jaguars eat the bark off the yaje vine to hallucinate.[32] Elephants make wine from palm sap.[33]

Birds fill up on fermented berries until they're drunk and disoriented enough to die by flying while intoxicated. Ducks seek out narcotic plants. Monkeys and dogs love opium smoke. Chimps will surmount their fear of fire to smoke cigarettes, and tobacco is addictive to a number of animals, including parrots, baboons, and hamsters. Reindeer will ignore food to pursue hallucinogenic mushrooms if they smell them in use by Lapp shamans.[34] Now consider that the poppy was one of the first domesticated plants—and ain't nobody harvesting those tiny little seeds to make a meal.

There are pharmacological substances in the annual domesticates called exorphins. They're opioids, affecting the human brain the way that opium does. And yes, they are addictive. Milk, another agricultural food, also contains exorphins, though in much lesser quantities. G. Wadley and A. Martin, the researchers who developed this theory, state,

> the ingestion of cereals and milk, in normal modern dietary amounts by normal humans, activates reward centres in the brain. Foods that were common in the diet before agriculture ... do not have this pharmacological property. The effects of exorphins are qualitatively the same as those produced by other opioid ... drugs, that is, reward, motivation, reduction of anxiety, a sense of well-being, and perhaps even addiction. Although the effects of the typical meal are quantitatively less than those of doses of those drugs, most modern humans experience them several times a day every day of their adult lives.[35]

According to Drs. Michael and Mary Dan Eades, "No one binges on steak or eggs or pork chops; they always binge on cookies and candies and other carbohydrate junk foods ... Cereal grains and products made from them have an allure that transcends the mere taste bud stimulation they provoke."[36]

We did it because we got addicted, because those annual grains offered up a happy, chemical hit. Plants have been playing with chemistry for one hundred million years, trying out strategies to repel potential predators and attract potential helpers. They make substances like caffeine that dull the appetite, hallucinogens that initiate massive confusion, hormones to disrupt future reproduction, and frank poisons to kill, all amazing in their precision. They also experimented with chemicals to attract, and that provide bliss, ecstasy, spiritual insight, and (all hail the goddess Theobroma) stimulate pleasure centers. Too much of this and the potential animal helper is a useless addict. But just enough and the addict can do a lot for the plant—and will do what it takes to get more.

Like conquer the world.

Start with a piece of land—a forest, a prairie, a wetland. In its native state the land is covered with a multitude of plants, working in concert with the microfauna—bacteria, fungi, yeasts—and with animals from insects to mammals. The plants are the producers, turning sunlight into mass, creating both the oxygen-rich atmosphere for the rest of us to breathe, and the topsoil on which the rest of us depend. This is called a *perennial polyculture. Perennial* because most of the plants live many years, sequestering carbon in their cellulose bodies, forming miles of vast root systems through the soil. *Polyculture* because there's so many of them, all cooperating, competing, contributing; all filling a niche with a necessary function. Perennial polycultures are how nature protects and builds topsoil, how life has organized itself to produce more.

This is what agriculture is: you take a piece of land and you clear every living thing off it, down to the bacteria. Then you plant it to human use with a tiny handful of species, often endless miles of a single plant like corn, soy, wheat. The animals are killed, often into extinction. They simply have nowhere to go. There were somewhere between 60 and 100 million bison in the United States in 1491. Now there are 350,000 bison, and only 12 to 15,000 of those are pure bison that were not crossbred with domestic cattle. The land held between 425,000 and a million wolves; only 10,000 now remain. Some species of ground-dwelling birds were wiped out before they even had names (European names, that is; I'm sure the indigenous peoples knew what to call them). The North American prairie has been reduced to 2 percent of its original size and the topsoil, once twelve feet deep, can now only be measured in inches.[37]

Agriculture is based on annual monocrops, the precise opposite of perennial polycultures, and it does the opposite of what nature does: it destroys topsoil. "The deterioration of the soil is the inescapable injury of agriculture to the environment," writes Steven Stoll.[38] Or as Tom Paulison puts it, "The planet is getting skinned."[39] Agriculture is a catastrophe that never allows the land to heal. And keeping the ground bare involves enormous effort. Because life wants to live. The trees keep trying to make a forest, the grasses want their prairie, and the waters ache for a wetland. Abandon cleared land in New England, and you'll get pokeberry and brambles, then sumac and birch, then maples and oaks and pines. In five years it'll be covered in saplings; in ten years they're too big to cut with a handsaw. This is the earth protecting itself, covering its body in a living armor of green.

But its armor isn't thick enough, not when the assailants are humans. Agriculture is more like a war than anything else, an all-out attack on the processes that make life possible. Daniel Hillel explains,

> by its very nature, [agriculture] is an intrusion and hence a disruption of the environment as it replaces a natural ecosystem with an artificial one ... The moment a farmer delineates a tract of land ... he is in effect declaring war on the preexisting environmental order. Wishing to grow a particular crop ... the farmer must now treat all the native species as noxious weeds or pests, to be eradicated by all possible means. However, in an open environment the wild species continue to reinstate their stolen domain, so the farmer's war is never finally won.[40]

Agriculture is a march to the sea that's encircled the globe. The only land left is the stuff agriculturalists can't use: too cold, too hot, too steep, too dry.

And agriculture isn't quite a war because the forests and wetlands and prairies, the rain, the soil, the air, can't fight back. Agriculture is really more like ethnic cleansing, wiping out the indigenous dwellers so the invaders can take the land. It's biotic cleansing, biocide. "In the history of civilization ... the plowshare has been far more destructive than the sword."[41] It is not non-violent. It is not sustainable. And every bite of its food is laden with death.

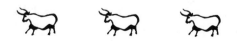

When I was in school, I took a class called "The Politics of World Hunger." I'd been a vegan for four years and I was well-versed in the solutions to world hunger. Or so I thought. It turns out I didn't know shit. The professor, an agronomist who also raised sheep, made a statement that sent a cold chill down my spine.

"The moment you put a plow to the soil, you degrade the soil."

I saw it all fall like dominoes, the whole human race. There were too many of us, billions too many, to use anything but agriculture to feed ourselves. Our numbers made us dependent on clearing land and using it for our species only. But that process was destroying the topsoil. Without soil, there'd be no food, no life. If what he was saying was true, the eventual end point was massive starvation.

"Plowing the soil exposes it to sun, rain, and wind," he explained. In case his words weren't clear, he had slides.

For example, he had pictures of Mesopotamia, the "land between the rivers", in what is now called Iraq. You might have seen the pictures—though probably from the perspective of reporters embedded with US troops, not agronomists trying to bring the desert back to life. The rivers in question are the Tigris and Euphrates. The area was named the Fertile Crescent, but no one in their right mind would call it that now.

> Wide stretches of barren, salt-encrusted terrain [are] criss-crossed with remnants of ancient irrigation canals. Long ago, these were fruitful fields and orchards ... The poor condition

... is due in large part to the prolonged exploitation of this
fragile environment by generations of forest cutters and burn-
ers, grazers, cultivators, and irrigators.... The once prosperous
cities of Mesopotamia are now *tells*, mute time capsules in
which the material remnants of a civilization that lived and
died there are entombed.[42]

The civilization of the Indus River Valley met the same fate.
India, Pakistan, Australia, Russia, the US, sub-Saharan Africa, Meso-
and South America, Egypt, Canada—if their arable land isn't already
salt-cracked, sun-baked clay, it will be. The Mediterranean, for instance, was once a forest. There actually used to be cedars in Lebanon,
not just the ghost of one on the flag. "The hills of Israel, Lebanon,
Greece, Cyprus, Crete, Italy, Sicily, Tunisia and eastern Spain" were
dense with trees and topsoil a meter deep.[43] Stripped of its protective
trees, the soil washed into the sea. All that's left now is scrubby brush
clinging to dry rocks browsed by goats, desiccating in the sun.

The city of Utica serves as an example of the scale of the destruction. Utica was a seaport at the mouth of the Bagradas River. But the
soil from the hills was carried to the sea by the river, where it built up
until Utica was no longer a port. The abandoned city now lies seven
kilometers from the coast, beneath ten meters of silt.[44] "The fate of
Utica," writes Daniel Hillel, "is typical of what has befallen the other
magnificent cities established by the Romans in North Africa."[45]

In Lebanon (and then Greece, and then Italy) the story of civilization is laid bare as the rocky hills. Agriculture, hierarchy, deforestation, topsoil loss, militarism, and imperialism became an intensifying
feedback loop that ended with the collapse of a bioregion that will
most likely not recover until after the next ice age. Lebanon was home
to the Phoenicians, the Mediterranean's premier sea traders. Their
arable land was circumscribed by mountains, on which cedars grew.
Cedar lumber is prized for building, and especially shipbuilding, as
it's naturally rot resistant. In case you think Maxxam and Plum Creek
invented it, the Phoenicians also clear-cut their land. Mesopotamia
and Egypt had no trees and were happy to buy. The Book of Kings
describes King Solomon sending laborers by the thousands to help

in the effort to cut and haul cedar timber back to Jerusalem, where it was needed ("needed") to build temples and palaces. Such buildings are a function of agricultural civilizations, with their hierarchies of kings and priestly classes.

Next, the exploding population tried to farm the sloped land, which led to the inevitable slide of soil into the sea. This led to the final stage of agriculture: imperialism. The Phoenicians colonized North Africa, Sardinia, Sicily, and Spain. The colonies provided food by mining their own topsoil, taking the Phoenicians' industrial products (mainly glass and dyes) in exchange.

Eventually Phoenician strength declined and the Greeks overtook them. In their turn, the Greeks destroyed their own lands, turning "a land once densely vegetated into a terrain of naked rocks."[46] They deforested for agriculture and for fuel for industrial processes like making pottery, bricks, and metals. They also used lumber for the construction of carts, chariots, and, of course, ships for trade and for the inevitable military conquests. The Greeks also burned their forest to make way for animal pasture, which they destroyed by overgrazing. Hillel quotes *The Iliad*: "Many a hillside do the torrents furrow deeply, and down to the dark sea they rush headlong from the mountains with a mighty roar, and the tilled fields of men are wasted." Warfare was the final insult to the land, as soldiers in the endless wars of the region would specifically cut down the trees of vanquished peoples. With the topsoil gone, there was no matrix to grow trees again.

The topsoil accumulated at the outlets of streams, eventually creating swamps. The swamps bred mosquitoes and the mosquitoes provided a vector for a brilliant new organism who found an unclaimed niche in the human blood cell. Malaria is a disease of civilization, one of the many. Writes Richard Manning, "[C]learing the tropical forest first in Africa, and later in ... other regions ... created precisely the sort of conditions in which mosquitoes thrive. Thus, malaria is an agricultural disease."[47] Every year between 700,000 and 2.7 million people die from malaria. Every minute, it kills two Africans.[48]

Then came Rome and the pattern repeated again: land cleared for agriculture and industry, topsoil washing away, rivers clogged at their mouths, streams running dry at their source. Explains Steven Stoll, "Topsoil holds most of the available water in any ecosystem. Without this reservoir, moisture finds the nearest watercourse; land dries out; climate changes."[49] Down at the bottom, the silt created more malarial marshes and destroyed the harbors at Ostia, Paestum, and Ravenna. Tracks of land, called *agri deserti*, or deserted fields, were left bare and abandoned. All powered by the toil and misery of human slavery.

> The Romans' mistreatment of nature was carried considerably beyond the environs of their own land. Everywhere they established their dominion, they repeated the same pattern. Forest clearing took place extensively, as did overcultivation and overgrazing of land to satisfy the avaricious demands of a bloated center of power.[50]

One could substitute the name of any bloated power center in place of Rome, and the same description of the agricultural juggernaut—environmental, economic, social—that has encircled the globe.

North America was once covered in forests so thick that a squirrel could theoretically travel from Maine to Texas without touching the ground. Where the rains gave out the prairies began, and grasses ran root to root for two thousand miles. There were rivers that swelled in their seasons, covering the land with a wild and tender flood of fertility, and wetlands that released the water like a long, slow sigh.

As I said, the native prairie is now 99.8 percent gone. Illinois was once swaddled in twenty-two million acres of prairie, with some forest groves and savannas.[51] In Nebraska, 98 percent of the native tallgrass prairie is gone.[52] There is no place left for the buffalo to roam. There's only corn, wheat, and soy. About the only animals that escaped the biotic cleansing of the agriculturalists are small animals like mice and rabbits, and billions of them are killed by the harvesting equipment every year. Unless you're out there with a scythe, don't forget to add them to the death toll of your vegetarian meal. They count and they died for your dinner, along with all the animals that have dwindled past the point of genetic feasibility. "You can look a cow in the eye," reads an ad for soy burgers. What about a buffalo?

Five percent of a species is needed to ensure enough diversity for long-term survival, and less than 1 percent of the buffalo are left.

Now, instead, we have agriculture. Indiana was once home to over two million acres of prairie and forest. Only a thousand fragmented acres are all that remain. There were also thousands of acres of tupelo gum and bald cypress swamps. Bald cypress are relatives of redwoods but no one does tree-sits to protect them. Tupelo gums are crucial to their animal cohorts, providing food for woodchucks, turkeys, bear, deer, fox, raccoons, squirrels, and many birds. They can live over five hundred years. There are a few small patches that have been alive since before Columbus. Survivors, indeed. The National Champion of Tupelo Gums—who knew?—was 105 feet high, with a 58 foot limb spread and a 27 foot, 1 inch circumference.[53]

Most trees suffocate under water. Their roots need oxygen. But tupelo gum and bald cypress grow a spongy tissue above the waterline, tissue that absorbs oxygen from the air like you and I do. "There's actual breathing going on," says Richard Hines, wildlife biologist at the White River National Wildlife Refuge.[54]

Maybe you don't find trees and grasses compelling as species. Maybe you don't think of them as sentient or suffering. But they are necessary for the creatures that do tug at your heart and conscience. The scale of what has happened on this continent—on this planet—is hard to absorb, especially when the knowledge brings nothing but grief for anyone who is still breathing. And to go even further, to question the nature of agriculture itself, is almost impossible. We live in an agricultural society. It feels like questioning air, or god, or progress, or human survival, personal and collective. We don't even know how to question it. We live, mostly, in suburban-urban areas long since decimated by saws and plows and abandoned to asphalt. We know what the books say—impassioned, compassionate books—with their hellish descents into factory farms and their righteous weighing of grain, all sixteen pounds. We don't know about black terns or Swainson's warblers or canvasback ducks. We have no idea who is dying to feed us.

We don't know what agriculture is because no one's ever told us and we can't see it for ourselves. We can't see it because the destruction has been so total we don't know what the world should look like. I've driven across Indiana four times and had no idea it was once part forest and swamp. Who would look at Indiana and think *swamp*? It wasn't until I read Gene Stratton-Porter's *The Girl of The Limberlost*— a children's novel about a determined girl who uses her knowledge of the swamp to pay her school fees—that I found out. The Limberlost swamp was 13,000 acres, protected by another 12,000 acres of wetlands. The Limberlost State Historic Site gets over 10,000 visitors a year, and two-thirds want to see the swamp. Becky Smith, the curator, has to tell each and every one, "The swamp does not exist."[55]

Soil, species, rivers. That's the death in your food. Agriculture is carnivorous: what it eats is ecosystems, and it swallows them whole.

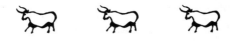

Could it be different? Is it the nature of agriculture or just the way we practice agriculture that's destructive? In that regard, is agriculture parallel to grazing? Appropriate animals integrated into perennial polycultures will add to the fertility—indeed, they are necessary for healthy woodlands, wetlands, savannas, and prairies. But too many animals or the wrong kind of animals will degrade the land, sometimes to the point of desertification. As discussed, white-tailed deer are destroying the northeastern forests because there aren't enough predators. Without wolves and mountain lions, there are more deer now than there were in 1491. Too-high stocking rates of cattle and goats are degrading land the world over. But that's not inherent in the nature of ruminants; the destruction comes not from doing it, but from doing it badly.

It is my conviction that growing annual grains is an activity that cannot be redeemed. It requires wholesale extermination of ecosystems—the land has to be cleared of all life. It destroys the soil because the soil is bared—and it *has* to be bared to grow annuals. In areas with inadequate rainfall, agriculture demands irrigation, which drains rivers to death and salinizes the soil. It also requires endless physical labor for sub-par nutrition. And it has devastated human cultures, leaving slavery, class stratification, militarism, population overshoot, imperialism, and a punishing Father God in its wake.

Has anyone been able to produce annual monocrops without the destruction? Can agriculture be sustainable?

Wes Jackson writes:

> Most of the northern European cultures and Japan have farms that are maintained in a seemingly sustainable way. But as we look at the success stories, we discover that a complex of factors exists, including the nature of the rainfall, the nature of the cropping system, the nature of the soils, and the nature of the culture, which combine in unique ways to promote a positively compelling sustainable agriculture. Even so, neither northern Europe nor Japan comes close to feeding itself. And the number of individuals or cultures that practice a sustainable agriculture that is positively compelling ... is small indeed. To suggest that the solution to the agricultural problem simply requires following the example of the ecologically correct around us today is a little like suggesting that if more people were like citizen Doe who displays good conduct, no police or military would be needed. Well, both the police and military do exist and both are signs of failure within and of civilization.... But should we not be constantly looking for ways to make them unnecessary? Should we not strive to create an agriculture which makes unnecessary the example of exemplary people within the current agricultural tradition?[56]

Two-thirds of the earth's land is unsuited for annual crops, destructive or not. It's simply too wet, too dry, too hot, too cold, or too steep to even try it. But where agriculture can be done, to approach soil sustainability, the rain has to be gentle and come fairly evenly across the warm season. The climate must also be temperate—too hot and wet, and the biological activity burns through the organic material quickly, leaving topsoil that's naturally too thin for agriculture (think rainforest). If the climate is too cold, then there isn't enough biological activity to degrade organic matter (think Greenland). The proper conditions are only matched in a few places on earth. Jackson mentions northern Europe and Japan. Note well the list doesn't include the major grain-growing regions of the world like the American Midwest. The summers are too hot, the rain too infrequent, and the storms too intense.

Beyond the climate and site factors, there's the cultivation practices. To approach soil sustainability, the fields are rotated from annual monocrops back to pasture—to animals on perennial polycultures—and then back to annual monocrops. The annual periods destroy the soil; the animals and perennials build it back. If you're very lucky the destruction and the rebuilding stay roughly even. But there is no way to do this without domesticated animals. A vegan agriculture is, in the words of Mark Purdy, an "ecological wasteland."[57]

Bill Mollison writes that nature builds topsoil at about 2-4 tons/ hectare a year, but in tilling we remove 40-500 t/ha a year. The worst-case scenarios of flood or bad winds can destroy *two thousand years* of soil in one season.[58]

What about non-tillage systems? They are effective at slowing topsoil losses. But to clear the land, the plow is replaced by herbicides. Do I really have to argue that spraying poison across continents is a bad idea?

So here is an agriculture without animals, the plant-based diet that is supposed to be so life-affirming and ethically righteous. First, take a piece of land from somebody else, because the history of agriculture is the history of imperialism. Next, bulldoze or burn all the life off it: the trees, the grasses, the wetlands. That includes all creatures great and small: the bison, the grey wolves, the black terns. A tiny handful of species—mice, locusts—will manage, but the other animals have to go. Now plant your annual monocrops. Your grains and beans will do okay at first, living off the organic matter created by the now-dead forest or prairie. But like any starving beast, the soil will eat its reserves, until there's nothing—no organic matter, no biological activity—left. As your yields—your food supply—begin to dwindle, you've got two options. Take over another piece of land and start again, or apply some fertilizer. Since the books, pleading and polemical, say that animal products are inherently oppressive and unsustainable, you can't use manure, bone meal, or blood meal. So you supply nitrogen from fossil fuel. Do I need to add that you can't produce this yourself, that its production is an ecological nightmare, and that one day the oil and gas will run out?

Your phosphorous will have to be made from rocks. There's a reason for the popular image that equates hard labor in prison with chopping rocks. How will you mine it, grind it, or transport it without fossil fuel, using only human musculature and without using slavery? For your potassium, you'll collect wood ashes, try some cover crops, and hope for the best. Meanwhile the soil is turning to dust, clogging the rivers, blowing across the continent. In 1934, the entire eastern seaboard was covered in a thick haze of brown, the topsoil of Oklahoma plowed to cotton and wheat, drifting like an angry ghost to cover the eastern cities and further, to ships hundreds of miles out to sea, a final, fitting tribute to the extractive economies of the civilized.[59] This is where agriculture ends: in death. The trees, the grasses, the birds and the beasts are gone, and the topsoil with them. More of the same is no solution.

Wes Jackson's answer is an agriculture based on perennial grasses. Right now, he's trying to domesticate perennials. He writes that "agriculture itself is an ecological problem outranking industrial pollution" and it's a problem he's devoted his life to solving.[60] He's attempting to breed perennial plants that will devote energy to seed production. Remember, one of the joys of being long-lived is there's time, time to develop roots and stems and woody mass, time to reproduce in a leisurely fashion. Perennial grasses don't produce large numbers of energy-dense seeds because they don't need to. Annuals, on the other hand, are on a schedule. From the moment they sprout, their biological clocks are ticking. Their survival strategy is big, fat seeds and lots of them. The question is, can the herbaceous perennials be coaxed into producing bigger seeds? "Some highly reputable plant geneticists I have asked, who have worked and thought on the question, not only have discouraging comments but lean toward a categorical 'no' when asked about the possibility of coexistence of perennials and high-yield," he reports.[61] Still, he's trying. But being a scientist, not a polemicist, his utopian farm of the future is still grazed by animals (cattle, buffalo, pigs, chickens) because animal manures are required by the soil. Those animals also eat the stuff we can't eat (cellulose stems) and turn it into stuff that we can (protein and fat).

Where I diverge from Jackson is in the *why*. Not the *why* of topsoil loss and annual monocrops. But the why of *why bother?* His goal is to develop an agriculture that functions like a prairie. My reply, which feels more like a plainsong, is that we already have prairies, or we did once. Humans have lived on savannas and grasslands for millions of years without devastating them, and without needing technical fixes. We shared them with other species and kept our own numbers at carrying capacity. We didn't destroy the world, our home. We need agriculture that functions like a prairie because our numbers have swollen past what the world can bear without us claiming more than our share of it. We have to turn actual prairies into shadow prairies because agriculture—especially the fossil-fuel based green revolution—has dramatically increased the human population.

Bill Mollison also has a solution involving the restoration of soil-building perennial polycultures, which he named "permaculture." He explains, "Even the most ideal tillage just keeps pace with the most ideal conditions of soil formation."[62] The best annual grain culture—given the correct climate, topography, and animal rotation—can only hope to replace what it's destroying. Not build, like nature does: only replace. And, yes, it's better to destroy less. I think the black terns must be pleading: please, destroy less. But why destroy at all?

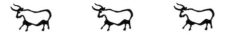

The mechanical destruction of clearing and plowing is destructive on its own, but a further problem is the salinization caused by irrigation. Dissolved salts are present in all irrigation water. While absorbing moisture, plant roots reject excess salt, because too much salt will kill the plant. The problem is that salts then start accumulating in the soil, and that build-up eventually reaches toxic levels. In areas where rainfall is plentiful, it may be sufficient to leach the salts through the soil below the root level. Of course, in those areas irrigation itself is probably unnecessary. It's the drier regions that will need irrigation and then won't have enough ambient rainfall to wash away the salts.

The problem is exacerbated by a rise in the water table "that, in the absence of adequate natural or artificial drainage, naturally follows the flood-irrigation of low-lying lands."[63] It can take years—generations, even—but eventually the water table gets close enough to the surface that evaporative capillary action starts. Now, as water evaporates off the surface of the soil, it pulls more water up from below, which then also evaporates. And all this water leaves salt behind. Think of a hot day, how your skin gets slightly sticky with salt from moisture evaporating off your surfaces. It's the same process. Desperate farmers across millennia have tried to save their land by applying more irrigation to flush salts out, but this only accelerates the problem by raising the water table higher.

Entire civilizations have collapsed as a result of doing this to their land, and the process is well underway in the major grain-growing regions around the world.

In case you need more convincing, I have in front of me a list of birds. Swainson's warbler is a small bird (5 to 6 inches) with a big voice. It pokes its bill inside fallen leaves to uncurl them in search of insects. "Condition at hatching," writes the Cornell Ornithology Lab, "helpless and naked."[64] The Acadian flycatcher can hover and fly backwards. The black tern with its gorgeous, glossy breeding plumage and its gregarious nature will live in flocks that can number in the tens of thousands—try to imagine the sky awash with twenty or thirty thousand birds. The male canvasback duck makes sweet coos when he's courting, and the female, like many bird mothers, pulls the down off her body to line her nest.

I won't belabor this. The list of birds is a roll call of the damned and it stretches from here to hell. And any bird dependent on a river will find its name written there.

Because I also have a list of rivers, rivers I've never even heard of, that are being destroyed for irrigation. They're being diverted and drained to grow crops like wheat, rice, and cotton, and also for industrial processes like hydro-electricity and dye works. "70% of all water from rivers and underground reserves is being spread onto ... irrigated land that grows one-third of the world's food," writes Fred Pearce, in *When the Rivers Run Dry*, a book that will break your heart. In "Egypt, Mexico, Pakistan, and Australia and across Central Asia, 90% or more of the water abstracted from the environment is for irrigation."[65]

Green revolution crops deliver more grain per acre, but in order to do it, they use more water. The water has to come from somewhere, and that means more dams, more wells, more diversion—and more salinization. Not only are we using nonrenewable fossil water—water from deep inside aquifers that recharge at a glacial speed if at all—but "projects that initially greened the desert are now creating desert."[66] Worldwide, 25 million acres of arable land are lost each year to salinization.[67]

Take Pakistan as an example. The Indus River supplies irrigation water for 90 percent of Pakistan's crops. (Keep in mind that very little grain is fed to animals in Asia and Africa—Chapter Three will address this more fully.) One hundred thousand acres each year are abandoned because of salinization. That's *one-tenth* of Pakistan's fields lost to date. Another fifth are waterlogged, and another quarter are barely producing.[68] Karachi is the fastest growing city in the world, exploding with a population of environmental refugees.

In some parts of the Sindh Province, over half the land is barren.

The Indus River, one of the original sites of civilization, now runs dry for its last few hundred miles. The delta of the Indus—and feel free to insert Mississippi, Ganges, Ebro, Yellow, or Volta here—was a species-dense series of wetland marshes, filled with fish, birds, and dolphins. But the march to the sea is happening in reverse. Without the silt that the river once carried, the delta is eroding. Without the barrier of a delta, the sea is encroaching. A million acres that were once mangrove swamps are now dead, drowned beneath the ocean.

Or take India. Two-thirds of India's crops are dependent on underground water. Wells in northern Gujarat once filled with water at thirty feet. Now wells at 1,300 feet run dry. Entire districts in Tamil Nadu and Gujarat are being depopulated. As the floods from the rivers fade, first into desert and then into myth, another flood takes their place: a flood of people from the countryside into slum-bloated cities.

Rice, wheat, corn—the annual grains that vegetarians want the world to eat—are thirsty enough to drink whole rivers. Countries dependent on green revolution crops have a water consumption rate several times that of Europe. Per capita, "Pakistan abstracts five times more water per person then Ireland does, Egypt five times more water than Britain, and Mexico five times more than Denmark."[69] Irrigation doesn't "just" destroy wetlands and riparian systems. As the water table drops, any trees left standing behind the plow die of thirst as their roots no longer reach water. All that's left is dust. And the dust builds into storms, spreading, for instance, from China's wheat fields across Asia, "choking lungs in Beijing, closing schools in Korea, dusting cars in Japan, and raining onto mountains and across the Pacific in western Canada."[70] The Yellow River begins in the plateaus of Tibet, in an area called "the county of thousands of lakes." Over half those lakes are only a memory on a map, having disappeared into wheat and rice below. The World Bank warns of the "catastrophic consequences" if China is unable to feed its people.[71] The rivers are also warning us, though they can't speak English. Of China's 23,000 miles of large rivers, 80 percent don't support fish anymore. If the earth could write a report, we would forgive it for using only two spare words: eighty percent.

Set aside the fossil fuel for the fertilizer and transportation. If you live in Burlington, Vermont or Santa Cruz, California, and you eat rice—ubiquitous, vegan brown rice—this is what you're eating: dead fish and dead birds from a dying river. It takes anywhere from 250 to 650 gallons of water to grow a pound of rice.[72] Pretend your rice was grown in North America. Picture Texas or California. They're dry grasslands of short-stem prairies. Or they should be. Now picture rice, tropically lush with green—and up to its neck in water. *Where does that water come from?* Now substitute "home" for "water": Long-nose gar and roseate spoonbills, American alligators and piping plovers. There's death on your plate, an entire ecosystem's worth, but it happened out past the asphalt, far, far out, in a world we will never know.[73]

Some of these projects are worse than others: wheat on the edge of the Gobi Desert (130 gallons of water/lb); rice in Sindh (250-650 gallons/lb); confinement dairy cows in the Sonora Desert (500 to 1,000 gallons of water for a quart of milk). Tony Allen, a water specialist, calls it "madness."[74] And it is. But the good and the bad are only different in degree, not kind. Damming rivers kills them. So, obviously, does draining them. Irrigation is bound to create salinization: like any conquering army, agriculturalists salt the land. Until what's left is asphalt and desert, variations on the theme called civilization.

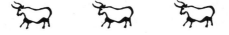

The Logone River in Cameroon gets its water from the Congo rainforest. The river and its floodplain have been the mainstay of hunters and fishermen, providing rich wildlife for millennia. The Fulani, the largest nomadic population in the world, have used the area for centuries. Then along came a state-owned rice company and its dam. The plan was to use the water to irrigate rice paddies. One dam and sixty miles of embankment later, the floodplain and its species-rich ecosystem were destroyed.

You could condense my entire book into the next two sentences.

"Rich pastures of perennial grasses died, so that some 20,000 head of cattle had to move away. Fish yields fell by 90%."[75]

Agriculture has wiped out everything in its path, including the humans. Considering this is Africa, they'd probably been living off some version of this pattern—ruminants on grass, fish from the rivers, *animals integrated into perennial polycultures*—for four million years.

We can round out the Cliffs Notes with three more sentences.

Meanwhile, elephants and lions in the Waza National Park, one of their last refuges in Central and West Africa, fled as their water holes dried up ... With the entire flood plain in crisis, the human inhabitants fought over water and pastures. Many left for distant cities.[76]

This sequence has been repeating itself for 10,000 years. The last people who know how to live sustainably—how to integrate themselves into the living landscape of grasslands and rivers—are pushed off by the agriculturalists, to disappear into a hostile world where, like the animals, they will surely die.

We are all these people, because in the end, none of us can live without grasslands and rivers, oceans and forests. Money, especially money accumulated into wealth, may buffer us for awhile. But the needle is almost on empty. We're out of topsoil, out of water, out of species, and out of space in the atmosphere for the carbon we can't seem to stop burning.

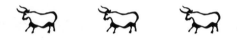

Then there's the Mississippi. Never mind the Indus and the Logone—realistically, most of us in the US couldn't draw those on a map. But the Mississippi runs through the heart of this continent, and in many ways, through the heart of this book. Only 2 percent of the US's rivers and wetlands are free-flowing. Less than half of the original wetlands remain.[77] Along the Mississippi and its tributaries, only 20 percent of the bottomland hardwood forests are left, and cut off from the rivers by levees, those are doomed to slow starvation.[78] Along with a final roll call of animals: canvasback duck, American crocodile (carries her babies to the water in her mouth), Hawksbill sea turtle, Louisiana black bear, gulf sturgeon. You don't need to hear the rest.

What you do need to hear is that the river has been destroyed for agriculture. To grow grain in areas with hot, dry summers requires water. Not a living river, but water. A real river floods. The wetlands luxuriate in silt and moisture, then slowly release the water back to the river. But agriculturalists want land. They take it from the forests and prairies and marshes, and they don't want it to flood. And once food is turned into a commodity, it has to be transported from where it's literally mined from the last of the dead prairie soils, to the population centers along the coasts from Portland, Oregon to Portland, Maine, and across the world. So the river is turned to water, confined to concrete channels cut deep enough for barges that carry the oil and gas to fuel all this, and for the barges that ship tons of annual grains that will become your daily bread. The channels stop the fresh river water from feeding the marshes and swamps—and the vacuum is filled by salt water. And digging deep enough for the barges also increases the flow of salt water entering marshes and swamps. The salt, of course, kills them.

Meanwhile snowmelts and heavy rain increase the volume and velocity of the water in the channels. Without wetlands to absorb the excess, the force of the water builds until the inevitable floods are catastrophic. Writes Ted Williams, "The only flood protection that ever worked is wetlands."[79]

When the water does finally explode into the Gulf, it's carrying a burden of nutrients—nitrogen runoff from row crops and factory-farmed animal manure—beyond what the normal balance of life-forms can absorb. The excess nitrogen causes algae to grow exponentially. As the algae die, the bacteria step up to the dinner plate. Now there's an abundance of bacteria, and they need oxygen. They need so much of it that nothing else breathing can live there. Anything that can swim fast enough gets out of the way. Anything that can't, dies. There is a dead zone at the mouth of the Mississippi that's the size of New Jersey.

Fertilizing with synthetic nitrogen leads to run-off because those fertilizers destroy the biological activity—the life—of the soil. Fertilizing with manure is ethically unacceptable to moral vegetarians, who consider domestication "exploitation," and to political vegetarians who think all arable land should be dedicated to growing annual grains. Desert and dead zones are the end point of an agriculture of annuals with no animals. Yes, the farms in the Mississippi watershed could apply fertilizer more sparingly. Please, apply it more sparingly. Maybe we can have a dead zone the size of Rhode Island instead. But is that really what you want to argue for?

Because here's the world I want.

> Before the US Army Corps of Engineers "improved" the river, as it likes to say, there were no floodwalls and levees for the Mississippi to blast through. It did not drown or render homeless the Americans who lived beside it and who simply moved their tepees when it languidly inhaled. On high ground they waited for the river to creep and seep through a rich mosaic of wooded islands, wild rice fields, sloughs, meadows, woods, ponds, and prairies—delivering seeds, renewing the earth with its gentle snow of sediments.
>
> With these annual inhalations came the floodplain spawners—bigmouth and smallmouth buffalofish and scores of others, depopulating drought-killed oxbows, easing through flooded timber and grasses, broadcasting eggs. Fry would fatten on plankton blooms, and in summer fingers of the gradually falling river would shepherd them back, leaving vast mud flats that fed migrating shore birds. Otters gorged on fish; cougars patrolled canebrakes; wolves hunted beavers in bottomland forests. On their spring and fall migrations ducks, geese, and other water birds streamed up and down the Mississippi's reach, resting and feeding in vast wetlands renewed by the unconfined river.[80]

And beside the river was a prairie that nurtured bison, antelope, grey wolves, and black-footed ferrets. And humans. We lived there once, too, not on it, but in it. We do have a choice, but it's not between life or death. It's between being predators or destroyers, between food that we live inside and food that we impose across the world.

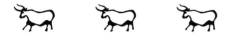

The Klamath refuge system is used by 80 percent of the migrating waterfowl along the Pacific Flyway. Klamath Lake hosts the biggest population of bald eagles in the continental US. The Klamath River was once the third most productive salmon river system in North America.[81] The salmon runs have been reduced over 90 percent. It's so bad for some species that they're considered endangered.

Salmon are called a keystone species.

> A keystone species is a species that has a disproportionate
> effect on its environment relative to its abundance. Such an
> organism plays a role in its ecosystem that is analogous to the
> role of a keystone in an arch. While the keystone feels the
> least pressure of any of the stones in an arch, the arch still
> collapses without it. Similarly, an ecosystem may experience
> a dramatic shift if a keystone species is removed, even though
> that species was a small part of the ecosystem by measures of
> biomass or productivity.[82]

In the case of the Northwest salmon, their spawning bodies bring a huge influx of nutrients to the other inhabitants of the river. They feed bears, otters, herons, eagles. Tons of nitrogen are embodied in the fish and distributed through the riparian community as the animals eat, digest, and defecate. Through this nutrient cycle, the fish feed the trees, and this is important because the trees are crucial to the life of the river. The trees provide shade which keeps the river cool enough for aquatic life. Trees store the water that comes as spring rain and snow melt, and then release it slowly as the ground slowly dries in warmer weather. This keeps water levels high enough to provide oxygen for fish. Fish feed trees, trees protect fish. Between fish and trees is a whole glissando of species from daphnia to eagles, and underneath them all is soil.

Beside the Klamath River is a long string of farms. Never mind that the region only gets twelve inches of rainfall a year—the river gives up its water for the farms. Thanks to the Klamath Irrigation Project, most of the water from the river basin in Oregon has been dammed and diverted for irrigation. In 2002, the water levels got so low that somewhere between 34,000 and 68,000 fish died.[83] They gasped and struggled and finally suffocated. Their bodies bloated and rotted, and I'm told the stench was unspeakable. This was done for the sake of agricultural products—potatoes, grain, onions—and for cattle.

Two months later I sat in a meeting at an activist conference. We were radical, righteous, and wrangling over food. The conference had served only vegetarian meals, but a growing number of us found that inadequate. Was there room for a range of options? No, because innocent animals shouldn't have to die. Meanwhile, in the kitchen, there was a whole shelf of lettuce in the fridge. Where was it grown? Who knows, besides far, far away. Probably California's Central Valley, where the waterbirds were once so thick over the Sacramento River that they blocked out the sun. But the river and its wetlands have been bled to death for agriculture, to grow lettuce, tomatoes, artichokes: non-violent, vegetarian, inherently more sustainable than animal source foods. Or such was the stand taken by my comrades.

And on the kitchen counter were three bags of potatoes, marked "Product of Oregon." No innocent rivers died for my food, I wanted to shoot back. But I am over thirty so I took a deep breath instead. It's not just what's dead on your plate, I tried to explain, there are way bigger questions you have to ask. Nobody wanted to ask them.

But this is my book, so I'll ask them here. What can feed humans on twelve inches of rainfall a year? Extend the question with the clause: without destroying such a brittle environment? A brittle environment with a river running through it? Why go through all the trouble of damming up and destroying a river, a river dense with fertility and food, and then all the work of planting onions and alfalfa and wheat, when you could just sit back and wait for the fish, year after year from now until forever? Is this insane, or is it just me? Cattle or other large ruminants like elk could eat the native grasses, though in much smaller numbers than thirsty alfalfa can support. Any attempt to grow annual crops, whether for animal feed or for vegetarian staples like wheat or soy, will destroy this land. It will, ultimately, destroy most land, but you'll see the results faster in an arid environment.

The moral vegetarians believe—and they believe it with all their hearts with all their good reasons—that the question is *life or death*.

But that is not the choice that nature offers any of us. We are all—apple trees and coho salmon, earthworms and black terns—predators, and then prey. *Life or death?* is not the question that will save us.

But this could be: what grows where you live? Ask it, and you'll see. To answer, you will have to know the place you live. And if your food, your survival, is dependent upon the place that starts at your beating heart and extends as far as your legs can walk in a day, you will have to learn about rivers and forests, soil and rain. Writes Derrick Jensen:

> If your experience ... is that your food comes from the grocery store (and your water from the tap), from the economic system, from the social system we call civilization, it is to this you will pledge back your life.... If your experience ... is that food and water come from your landbase ... you will make and keep promises to your landbase in exchange for this food.... You will be responsible to the community that supplies you with food and water. You will defend this community to your very death.[84]

What grows where you live? means what can grow, what should grow, who should grow it? And for all of us it means: who is destroying the place where you live? Corrupt or even totalitarian governments? A political dictator? A sociopathic economic system that turns corporate boards into legal persons with no responsibility to anything except shareholder profits? Coal or timber companies? The triumvirate of oil, auto, and construction industries that is literally paving the road to hell? The World Bank? Or are there simply too many people to ever eat sustainably from your foodshed? Over one hundred countries depend on grain from Canada and the US, and that grain constitutes 60 percent of all exports. For that matter, Massachusetts imports 85 percent of its food. The last time Massachusetts was self-sufficient for food, there were half as many people—and the land was 90 percent deforested, so we've got a problem.[85] Because there are too many people for the land—any land—to support, we consistently face Hobson's choices: do we grow as much as we can locally and destroy the local landbase, or do we import, and destroy somewhere else?

So *What grows where you live?* becomes *Why are there so many of us?* This leads into the question of who controls women's bodies. Those of us who actually are women? Or are women just another resource for men to use, in their endless quest to prove their toxic masculinity and breed soldiers for civilization's constant state of war? The masculinity and the war—against people, against the planet—together have created a perpetual motion machine of domination and destruction of the land and human rights. We will need to stop both to save this planet. This is why militarism is a feminist issue, why rape is an environmental issue, why environmental destruction is a peace issue.

Those are all huge spin-outs from the same beginning place of objectification, the process of turning living beings into things. The rain, the river, the long stem grasses—are they members of your community? Do you live inside your foodshed, or is the living land just topsoil to be used until it's dust? Are your human neighbors in other countries participants in a common project of care and connection, or are they labor units to assemble your cell phones, and how many soldiers will it take to keep them assembling? If you are a man, do women exist to make you dinner and sons? If you are a woman, you must surely burn for more. And for all of us, the planet is dying under civilization's regime: what will it take for us to fight back?

What grows where you live? One small question that could save the world.

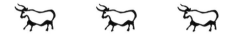

At this point in my education, the desperate vegan in me had to concede the following: Agriculture isn't possible on two-thirds of the world's land. It's too cold, too steep, too wet, too dry. My answer to this: fine, then people shouldn't live there. That I lived in one such place—New England, with its cold, rocky hills of thin, acid soil—was bracketed out of consciousness. "New England was naturally forested and agriculture was never appropriate for very much of this land," I read and promptly forgot.[86]

I also conceded that growing annual monocrops in the places it was possible would destroy the soil eventually. I answered this with a prayer to Wes Jackson, hoping that he'd be successful in my lifetime, and a vague plan to grow a lot of nut trees when my longed-for farm materialized.

I conceded that irrigation was indefensible. I had no problem there. If it meant a smaller human population, well, we had to get to work on lowering our numbers and raising the status of women.[87]

I conceded that I would need domesticated animals—their labor and the products of their bodies—to farm sustainably. I needed their manure and their unspeakable bones, their inconceivable blood. I slipped back and forth across a very narrow ethical line, aghast at my own willingness to even consider participating in domestication, which was by definition the exploitation of animals. How could I stop the insects that were after my food? Chickens and ducks were the permaculture answer, in complete opposition to the vegan answer. And what about the fertilizer? Maybe I could find another source of unused manure. Well, maybe I could, but that's like suggesting dumpster diving as a solution to economic oppression. I'd only be skimming the excess and pretending. The basic fact remained: some-body had to keep those cows and goats so I could use the manure. Animals, exploited for milk, meat, and eggs, were necessary for my food, whether I kept or ate them or not.

Maybe—I inched toward the side of evil—maybe I could have them without exploiting them. I could adopt animals nobody want-ed—old hens, boy goats—let them live out their natural lives, and in exchange I could have their manure and their bug-eating services. All right, fine, it was a compromise, dependent on meat and milk. But the animals were already *here*. And they didn't have to *die*. Did they?

Because lots of other things did. I was locked in mortal com-bat with the slugs. In dry years, they damaged the garden. In rainy years, they devastated it. I'd plant starts that were eaten to the ground twenty-four hours later. Poison was out of the question. It would kill and keep on killing the million and one microbes I was trying to encourage, the birds, the reptiles, bioaccumulating up the food chain, spreading another shadow of cancer and genetic damage across a darkening planet. So I tried an organic solution: diatomaceous earth. It worked. In two days the garden was slug-free and the lettuce was mine. Then I found out how it worked. Diatomaceous earth is the ancient bodies of small, prehistoric critters ground into powder. Each grain of powder has tiny, sharp edges. It kills by mechanical action. Soft-bellied animals like slugs crawl across it and it slices a million cuts into their skin. They die from slow dehydration.

I was horrified by what I'd done, and horrified more that I hadn't known. Where was the outrage? There was enormous overlap between vegetarian and organic proponents, both residing under a rough progressive-to-radical sustainability banner. There was a vague Everybody who knew that veal meant torture, that herbs were the people's medicine and could cure anything, that Oreos contained lard.[88] Mollusks are animals: why didn't anyone care?

And for one second, I knew the answer: slugs couldn't scream.

Copper barriers repelled slugs, but I couldn't afford those. I tried the really woo-woo stuff: I prayed, I sang, I burned sacred herbs from continents near and far, I left offerings, I pleaded with the Great Slug Mother. But the lesser slugs didn't care. They wanted to eat, and I couldn't blame them.

So I tried handpicking. I set the alarm to the middle of the night and stumbled out into the dark where the cold dew soaked right through my vegan canvas sneakers. I picked and picked and picked. I slowed the rate at which they were winning, but they still won. And the next morning I had a plastic container full of slugs. What now? Was there a Farm Slug Sanctuary somewhere? I'd wedge my feet back into my still-damp sneakers, hop on my bike, and ride down to where the houses ended and a little stretch of woods began. And? I know: the suspense must be killing you. I let them go. Which, as you can imagine, took a wee bit longer than releasing, say, a squirrel. Eventually they all slimed their way to freedom. But the wait gave me time to observe, and to let the observation swell into knowledge: there wasn't much for them to eat here. Not compared to my garden. Two plus two equals ... That's why there *were* so many in my garden.

And here? They were going to starve. This small patch of trees already had all the slugs it could use. That's what nature does: it fills every niche. If there's a free lunch, somebody eats it. In that quiet little space of trees, adult knowledge began to fill me like a slow river. Slugs—these slugs or other slugs—were going to die, and they were going to die so I could eat. But the trees weren't tormented by that fact, or not that I could tell. The silence of the woods, of the long seep of time through trees and leaves and rot and trees again, was its own prayer. And it wasn't a prayer of repentance, but a prayer of thanksgiving.

If the slugs had to die, then I had to be honest. I had to face it. My food—my life—was supposed to be about integrity and courage. If I had to kill—swallow hard, lift chin—to kill something, then at least I would do it with as little pain as possible. Diatomaceous earth took two days. Surely there was something quicker.

Beer. Slugs love it. They drink until they're drunk and then they drown. At least they die anesthetized and happy. I got a big bottle of something cheap and left little containers of it scattered about the salad greens. I went to bed steely with resolve: tonight, I was killing.

And I woke up at 2 AM in a panic. I couldn't do it. On went the sneakers, in went the dew, out went the beer. If I had to give up my garden for the year, well, at least I wasn't killing.

A week later, I was forced into the produce aisle at the grocery store, still relieved that I hadn't killed. With my clean, vegan hands, I picked up a head of lettuce.

Who the fuck are you fooling? may have been the first words of my adult life. Like the people growing that lettuce didn't kill slugs? Or if they didn't, of what possible value was food grown on land so eviscerated by industrial farming that it supports no other life besides chemically-coddled lettuce?

And not just slugs. Rabbits, raccoons, groundhogs, deer. I knew what my food was up against. There in the produce aisle, vegetarian, vegan even, I knew there was no escape. Death lay in the red burst of peppers, in the pregnant sweetness of the melons. It waited behind the sturdy green of the broccoli and it protected the soft tenderness of the lettuce.

And I hedged one more time. Okay, the slugs had to die, but I still wouldn't kill. I would get chickens and ducks and they would kill. For me? No, it was their nature, their instinct to hunt insects. And death by ducks was quick, quicker than diatomaceous earth. As quick as, well, nature had decided. Wasn't death natural?

Was it? Or wasn't it? Which way did I want the answer to fall?

Because if death was natural—a part of life, not an insult to life—*then why was I a vegan?*

I didn't go there. I went instead to the chapters in my homesteading books on fowl. I agonized and I mulled and I prevaricated. I also moved in with someone who had a house on five acres, two of meadow and the rest maple and pine forest. The farm could begin.

Eventually twenty-five baby chicks arrived, a box of cuteness made flesh. Never mind Trollope's baby worship. Chick worship consumed me. I lost hours just staring. They were the joy of my days. The next year they were joined by ducks and geese, then by guinea fowl and pigeons. And it was their nature to do the tasks I needed. They ate bugs. The chickens, in fact, ate anything that moved: mice, frogs, snakes. I once found a chipmunk tail in their yard: just the tail. I've seen them chase squirrels, which was funny until it dawned on me that if they were smart enough to hunt in packs they could take down a squirrel. In fact, the subject-object position of "humans eat chickens" might well be reversed. They pretty much ate anything I didn't want to, and they ate plenty of stuff I flat out couldn't, like grass. I'll never forget the first day I brought Miracle, my little duck, into the garden with me. I didn't have to teach her. She knew. One bite of bug and she exploded into quacks of joy: *this is what I was born for!* The slugs were history. And I wasn't killing.

Neither was Eichmann, whispered the Vegan Voice of Truth. Was this a death camp for animals, the furred, feathered, exoskeletoned? But everything seemed so peaceful. The birds were so obviously happy, looking for bugs.

Sure, and Arbeit Macht Frei. All Eichmann did was arrange the transportation. Isn't that what you've done?

But I have to eat something, I begged, stretched to the end of my ethical rope. *Something. Right?*

But beyond the spare shore of the vegan world lay the hungry sea of the fruitarians and the voyage out led to the promised land of the breatharians—people who believed that humans in fact don't need to eat.

I had met a few of them on my vegan pilgrimage. They radiated an intense fixation on food. When could they eat again, and how little/how much was the axis they were stretched across. The torturer or the tortured?

I remember Starling and her half-cup of yogurt, exactly half, once a day. A banana for breakfast, the smidgen of yogurt at noon, an apple at 4:00 PM. She'd been "weaning" herself from food and was aiming for pure air in another six months. Watching her eat was like watching an athlete, the exact balance between effort and discipline. Would she take an extra bite? Lick the drop that hung on the bottom of the serving spoon? Or would she force herself to perfection, to stick the landing, to achieve the supremacy of will and its reward, the grace of effortlessness? That's where anorexia ends, the pure physiology of starvation: the body stops wanting food, though I didn't know that then. There was something in Starling's project that I wanted, too: that grace, beyond need and hunger, beyond death. If getting there felt more like punishment, I was willing to endure it, if the goal was just and noble enough.

So how noble was this goal? Looked at through my vegan eyes, it was a possible end point of my desperate urge to refrain from killing. Why even kill plants when I didn't have to kill at all? But looked at through my feminist, political eyes, I was uneasy about this project. Religions around the world engaged in ascetic practices like severe fasting, and what those religions had in common was patriarchy. Their He-God was removed from the earth, and holiness was achieved by denying the world, made of flesh. Women were temptations of sin, our bodies sources of shame instead of miracles. "To live without eating was, of course, to deny one's need for material support or earthly connection," writes Joan Jacobs Brumberg in *Fasting Girls: The History of Anorexia Nervosa*.[89] The pagan in me rebelled against the idea of vilifying hunger, sex, bodies—life. Was there a way to starve without starving, to embrace life so fully I could live on air, light, energy, the cosmos? Anything besides dead things?

I had two competing impulses, two political belief systems that went to my core and conflicted. At twenty-six, the practical won out: I knew I had to eat. Even as a teenager I'd been bad at dieting. I couldn't embrace hunger—it was too miserable, and I always ended up binging. So I set aside Starling and her sip of communion yogurt, and all my questions about bodies and god and grace. I was a vegan. That was righteous and it was enough.

Except now I was arranging for animals to be killed, killed for my benefit. My personal Auschwitz. Maybe it was time to revisit the breatharians. In the interim, Al Gore had invented the internet, so the research was easy. I found Peter the breatharian, 5' 9" and 115 pounds. He was so proud of himself that he posted pictures. It was ghastly. Do I need to actually say that he was starving? He had links to pro-ana websites and trigger pix to help you keep your eating disorder firmly enshrined. He offered to teach you how to break your addiction to—no, not self-hatred—food. "Do you throw up?? If no, would you be open to this option?"[90]

Okay, I didn't need to go any further into his happy, healthy world. But what about the other articles, the ones that hinted at mystic possibilities? Jasmuheen (Ellen Greve) claimed, "I can go for months and months without having anything at all other than a cup of tea. My body runs on a different kind of nourishment."[91]

Australia's *60 Minutes* arranged to observe her. Dr. Berris Wink, president of the Queensland branch of the Australian Medical Association, made her stop the test after four days. Her speech had slowed, her pupils had dilated, and she was "quite dehydrated, probably over 10%, getting up to 11% ... Her pulse is about double what it was when she started. The risks if she goes any further are kidney failure."

Then there was the founder of the Breatharian Institute of America, with the rather fitting name of Wiley Brooks. He claimed he had been a breatharian for thirty years. In 1983 he was spotted leaving a 7-Eleven with hot dogs and Twinkies. He admitted that he sometimes broke his fasting with a Big Mac and a Coke. He explained that since he was surrounded by junk food, consuming it added balance. How's that for a new Twinkie defense?

Then there were the people who'd died: Verity Linn, kindergarten teacher Timo Degen, Lani Marcia, Roslyn Morris. Jim Vadim Pesnak and his wife Eugenia went to jail for three years for their involvement in Morris's death.

But Hira Ratan Manek said he could live on water supplemented by the occasional cup of tea, coffee, and buttermilk. He was under observation for three long fasts. During those fasts, however, he did lose a lot of weight. The papers published on these fasts also admitted that dozens of people had access to Manek during the studies, and the studies themselves would never have met western scientific standards.

Prahlad Jani also claimed to be a breatharian, though *The Indian Rationalists* labeled him a "village fraud." But the literature is filled with intriguing hints for anyone prone to believe. Practitioners of Chinese Qigong and other mystical traditions make all sorts of claims. The credulous and the desperate have plenty of material to work with.

Case in point. "Sweetie, um, do you think..." I stumbled. Saying something out loud always makes it more real. I managed to get to the word "breatharian."

"Lierre," replied my beloved, in that tone of patiently suppressed exasperation that I've forced her to perfect, "it's called *anorexia*. And," she continued, emphasizing each word, just to make sure, "if you try it, I'm leaving."

The voice of reason can be such a relief to people like me.

"But the ancient mystical Tibetan..." I tried, fervently hoping she'd be able to stop me.

"Okay, let's pretend it's true. Is it really the best use of your life to travel to Tibet in search of some guy on some mountain so you can learn *not to eat*? Is that really what you want to do with the time you've been given?"

On balance, no. Saving the world seemed like a better To Do list. I was free.

But in exchange, I had to accept death. Besides the slugs, there were other things that had to die, so many other things, and all of them had mothers and faces, if I looked. Information was becoming knowledge, knowledge I had missed because there was simply no one to tell me. I was taught to look both ways before crossing the street. I learned how to read when I learned to talk. I was even in on the secret of where babies came from. I remember at five earnestly explaining the word "vagina" to another little girl. I didn't know the word "empowerment," but that was my impulse. But food? That was a knowledge gap I didn't close until I was almost forty, and only after battling myself into emotional, physical, and ethical exhaustion.

So I had twenty-five chickens. The dead insects I could still play moral hide-and-seek with. But twenty-five hens meant twenty-five dead roosters. Here's why.

Animals may reproduce in 50/50 sex ratios but they don't necessarily live that way. A common pattern is that males reach maturity and engage in dominance battles until the excess males are killed or driven out. These are the hard facts: to be driven out is to die. Chickens typically live in groups of about twenty hens with one or two cocks. This has nothing to do with humans. It's how the species Chicken has organized itself. The roosters fight until most of them are dead or gone. Gone where? Into the stomach of a predator.

And that would be us.

It's cruel to force extra roosters into a flock, cruel to the hens. They'd have open bloody scrape marks down their backs from being mounted too frequently. I'd call that animal abuse. So what was I supposed to do with the extra males? I tried keeping the hens and roosters separate, but the boys spent their days pacing along the fence trying to get in with the girls. In their spare time, they inflicted grievous bodily harm on each other. The noise was unbearable. I hate to imagine substituting bulls for roosters. That was my first year of chickens, under the banner "Eggs, not meat!" I was desperate to draw lines, and to keep myself firmly on the moral side. In the end I found homes for two of the best roosters, a Black Australorp and an Araucana. And the rest? I gave them to a family down the street, a family who raised meat birds. Were my hands clean? As long as I didn't look down at them. My land needed chickens. Some of those chickens needed to die. Whether or not I ate them, for my food to be sustainable and organic, some animals had to die. I tried buying only hens from the hatchery, but I already knew the information I was running from. If I buy twenty-five heirloom hens, there's twenty-five baby brothers that nobody wants. Because nobody wanted those roosters. The hens were one, two, three dollars each. The roosters they couldn't give away. People raising their own broilers bought chickens known as Cornish x Rocks, which have been bred for meat production.[92]

So, I found out, the heirloom rooster chicks were killed. They were turned into pet food or farm and garden fertilizer. Which is to say that they were either eaten by your pets or, after a pass through a plant, you.

Please do not suggest that I should have "liberated" the roosters in the woods somewhere. People dump animals all the time in rural areas. They die. They starve or get eaten by predators. It's much kinder and more honest to kill them. At least as a human you can do it quickly.

And if they don't die, if they manage to establish themselves, congratulations. You've just introduced an invasive exotic to take over the niche of a native species, probably another ground-dwelling bird that's holding on by its claws. The feral pig is one domesticated animal that has been able to thrive in the wild, and they're destroying ecosystems in places like Hawaii. The native plants and animals have no defenses against them, especially their destructive rooting habits, and they have no predators, no check on their numbers.

Here's the portion of the birds and bees talk that urban industrialists, including vegetarians, seem to have missed along the way. Animals reproduce. And here's the math lesson to go with it. If you've got ten acres and ten cows, next year you'll have twenty cows, twice what your land can carry. Assuming half the new calves will be male, you've got fifteen females and five males. The following year you'll have thirty-five cows, 3.5 times your land's carrying capacity. By then the pasture will have eroded to dirt and everyone will be starving.

So you've got two problems. There will always be excess males. Of course on most farms that isn't a problem, because the point of the endeavor is food, and "meat" is not a four-letter word. Farm people eat the roosters as well as the male mammals. But there will also be excess females. For dairy animals to lactate, they have to bear young every year. A dairy cow should have a milking life of twelve to fourteen years. That means she'll have about eleven calves. Only one is needed to replace her. And the other ten? Where do you think veal comes from? That's why I was a vegan, not a vegetarian. That's why vegans call milk "liquid meat." And I can't tell you the number of vegetarians who, over the years, have refused to believe me. Simply, stalwartly, refused.

"Go ask a dairy farmer" is my final attempt.

But of course, they don't know any.

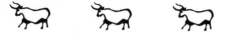

I've been to farms that were balanced on the vegan/sustainable tightrope. They all have fowl: chickens, ducks, guineas. "It's a compromise," they invariably say, always defensive. The other visitors are puzzled. Compromise? Don't chickens live on farms? And don't farms need chickens? It's only a compromise if you're trying to overlay a vegan ethic onto the biological truth of soil and the nutrient cycle. It's those facts that leave vegans with a Little Farm of Horrors and plants demanding *feed me!*

I spent a weekend at one of those farms for a conference on reviving local economies. It was in upstate New York. The directions to the place were essentially "drive to Canada, turn around." It was cold even in August. They said they were vegan and they said they did permaculture. What I saw was an uneasy hybrid, and like all hybrids, it was ultimately sterile. They had a lot of perennial beds, full of fruit trees, vines, and shrubs, piled deep with mulch and roped off. "Do not walk on beds," signs entreated everywhere.

"Please don't walk on the beds," repeated Doug, a man so emaciated that when I first met him, my heart was punctured by compassion. *Cancer—chemo—oh god,* was my first reaction. But he wasn't dying. He just wasn't eating. The interns—young, earnest, committed—looked about as bad. Some of them had a noticeable C curve in their posture, too much muscle wasting to stand up straight. A few of them were completely zoned out; it wasn't from pot, since the land was drug-free, so I had to conclude it was a starvation high. Was I the only one who noticed? Was everyone else that numb to a skeletal aesthetic?

"We're a permaculture site," he explained. "We don't till or plow. We're building soil with mulch and, except for some annual vegetables, they're all perennials."

So far, so good.

Asian pears, gooseberries, hardy kiwis, blueberries. It's all nice stuff, but humans can't live on fruit. What were they eating?

Around the back were the chickens and guineas.

"We need them for pest control and to clear garden beds," he apologized. Theoretically. In fact, the birds were in a wire pen, and while they had plenty of room and a nice secure house, they had long ago scratched the earth bare. No grass, no bugs: what were *they* eating?

The economic mainstay of the farm was the trees. "Trees are what we have," he defended. "Look at this land. See the slope? The soil? We can barely grow lettuce." So they did sustainable logging, wood products. And that meant a pair of draft horses. More apologies. Unlike tractors, horses required no fossil fuel, no steel mills or extractive mining, no bank loans. They can heal themselves, and they reproduce. But what were *they* eating?

Past the horse barn were a few acres that had been clear-cut to stumps. Two pigs and two goats were, finally, eating.

"We need these animals to clear this land for us," Doug pleaded. The goats were does, but he was quick to add that he wasn't going to breed them. I could see they were Nubians—dairy goats—the Jersey cows of the caprian world. What kind of sense did any of this make, these moral bargains against the facts of life? Because life was not going to meet Doug halfway.

The land was being cleared to make pasture for the horses. Right now they had to buy hay from another farm. All right, one loop closed: the horses would be fed.

Then the dinner bell rang, a gong that sang like gold across the mountainside. It was beautiful there, the hills the green of deep summer, gentled with sun. Fifty people lined up outside the dining hall, hungry. What we ate was bread and lettuce.

We repeated this meal six times over the next forty-eight hours. Breakfast was mostly pancakes, though it included a spare spoonful of scrambled eggs for the less-evolved, dished out with an expression of smug pity. "No eggs, no dairy!" the sign above the pancake griddle celebrated. Sure. How many times over how many years did I gnaw my way through such culinary delights? Lunch was bread and salad. Dinner was bread baked into a casserole with soy milk, and vegetable soup Dickensian in its lack—and please, sir, I did not want some more. Sunday was a breakfast of bread and a lunch of bread. They were proud of this bread, baked in an oven of handmade bricks, Doug explained, and fired by wood they harvested themselves. All commendable. Life-support that starts from the question: how can I live here without hurting this land? How can I take what I need without destroying?

But the food itself? The question hit the wall of ideology, and ideologies can build a sizable wall, as Berlin can well attest. Here were people so committed to their topsoil that they roped off five acres of garden beds. They certainly understood the principle of following nature's template: soil covered at all times in perennial polycultures and permanent mulch. But the basis of their diet was wheat and soy, annual monocrops grown out of the last biomass of the decimated prairie two thousands miles away. This farm was afloat on the Mississippi River and the Ogallala aquifer.

The only thing standing in the way of true sustainability was their vegetarianism. Because they could easily have been self-sufficient for food. The goats and pigs were already on site, already eating food that actually grows in upstate New York. If they'd bred the does and the sows, and let the fowl reproduce, they would have had a supply of meat, milk, and eggs that would have lasted from now until the sun burns out. Instead, there was essentially no protein on the table, or on the people for that matter. The only fat was optional. The butter (a concession, I'm sure, but the other choice is hydrogenated oil) was from Wisconsin, organic but insane when three hundred yards away there were two healthy mammals, filled up on forest browse, ready and willing to lactate. There was also olive oil for the salads. Sure, the Canadian border is a region renowned for its olive trees.

And the salads? The lettuce, at least, was grown on site, fertilized by the fowl manure, even though the birds were also surviving on the corpse of the prairie. The fowl ate almost nothing but grain, supplemented by occasional weeds and scraps thrown over the fence. The purpose of these birds remains a mystery, their contribution a net loss. They weren't allowed out to forage for greens and small animals. All their food had to be purchased. Nobody would admit to wanting their eggs, and the eggs of fowl fed such an unnatural diet are nutritionally deficient.[93] They certainly weren't being raised for meat. I was a guest in Doug's home, and there was only so much I could ask, so to this day I still don't know the purpose of the birds.

Sunday's salad was a big bowl of raw kale sprinkled with nasturtium flowers. You know those nightmares where you're back in junior high and you have to start over because you missed a gym class? And at some point you start to remember, wait! I have a job, a house, a Ph.D., an eight-year-old child. You cling to whatever symbols of adulthood you've accumulated—*they can't make me do this*—to try to wake up?

Staring down at the plate of raw kale, I woke up. They couldn't make me go back. They couldn't make me eat this. I'd done enough damage to my body—my thyroid, my joints—by eating the inedible. For twenty years I'd choked down some frankly disgusting food, and I'd made myself like it. No more. I scraped my plate into the compost bucket and I didn't care who saw me. And I rejoiced. I had firmly and forever left that world where starvation was the standard and politics a thin gruel of nourishment.

And on the eight hour drive home? My carpool begged to stop for pizza and ice cream, and we soaked up animal protein and fat like parched ground in the rain.

Again: for someone to live, someone else has to die. A friend offered that to me once, and it helped. This was the ancestral wisdom of her people. I don't have an unbroken line back to a living, pre-agricultural tradition, but the fragments that survive whisper to a similar theology.

In the animist world view, everything is alive: rocks, rain, rivers, birds. According to Luther Standing Bear:

> From Wakan Tanka, the Great Spirit, there came a great unifying force that flowed in and through all things—the flowers of the plains, blowing wind, rocks, trees, birds, animals—and was the same force that had been breathed into the first [human]. Thus all things were kindred... [94]

Here, there is no hierarchy where humans and maybe a few animals like us are the beings that count as "sentient," or "conscious," or somehow more worthy. We are all made of the same substance, a substance animate and sacred. Because of that similarity, because we are all siblings, communication with plants, animals, stars, and even the dead is an accepted and expected activity. The animating substance is more energy than mass, more motion than thing. It passes through us, temporarily taking the form of a fish or a flower, and then it's transformed into a heron or a hummingbird, and then again into a coyote or an apple. And even though fish and flowers die, Fish and Flowers continue. Jessica Prentice, the mother of the word *locavore*, explains:

> In ancient Greek, for example, there were two different words for "life": *bios* and *zoë* ... [A]ll living things rely on the death of other living things ... *zoë*-life, life in the biggest sense of enduring life, Life with a capital L, requires the sacrifice of *bios*-life, the particular lives of living creatures. *Zoë* takes (kills, consumes, eat, sacrifices, requires) *bios*. A core understanding of this adult knowledge lies at the heart of many spiritual practices and religious traditions worldwide. Death extin-

guishes a particular life, of course, but it doesn't extinguish
Life. Life endures and transcends death.[95]

And the beauty in this is that, nice as it would be to have a wise,
ancient grandmother to teach us, we don't have to have one. All we
need to do is observe. Find a small wild spot somewhere, the edge of
a parking lot, the tree outside your window, and watch. Really watch.
This is what you will see: everything is eating and then being eaten,
and through it all life endures. There is no hierarchy, only hunger.
And it's through our hunger that we participate in the cosmos, in an
endless cycle of life, death, and regeneration. For 98 percent of our
time on Earth this was our religion.

The religions of the civilized are equally similar. Gore Vidal calls
them "the Sky God people."[96] God is removed from the living world
(and changes gender), leaving the earth defined as inert matter. The
sacred is reduced to a punishing Father, split from all life processes.
The only thing holy is far above—and you disobey Him at your own
peril. Morality is a rigid code, the one true way, not a lived experience. The further humans move (or are moved, often by force) from
hunters to horticulturalists to agriculturalists to urbanists to industrialists, the further the sacred recedes, first to heaven, then condensed
to monotheism, until finally it dies in irony.

In one sense, humanism was simply the last step in the process
of desacralization. Man dispenses with the sacred altogether, putting
himself at the center of the moral universe. And in some ways this is
an improvement. Personally, I would rather live in a liberal democracy
than a religious theocracy. Funny how little things like voting and,
say, being able to leave the house without a male relative's permission,
matter. But religious theocracies are the result of agriculture. That
level of organized hierarchy didn't exist until civilization.[97] And I recognize fully that human rights have been won only at the cost of generations of struggle and that we aren't finished yet. Just for instance,
there are 27 million people still enslaved around the world, including
1.3 million women and girls bought and sold into sexual slavery.

But the narrative of capital-P Progress reads a little too much like
the story of Manifest Destiny or God dispensing Promised Lands. Be-

cause while we—human race we—have made theoretical and material strides toward a single, universal standard of human rights, we've also lost in ways that are crucial to the survival of life on earth.

The ancient world of the West saw the earth and the cosmos as a living body, and even into Christian Europe there were still religious strictures against human harm to the earth. But humanism removed those last restraints on human activity by killing off God, and replacing the metaphor of a body with that of a machine.[98] The world has been dying at an exponential rate ever since. Kinda hard to call that progress.

Humanism leaves us a contradictory legacy. In some ways it is an unfulfilled promise: all people should have the rights guaranteed by documents like the United Nations Universal Declaration of Human Rights. At least humanism gives us an ethical platform to argue from. If all men are created equal, then "all" can't just mean "white and rich" and "men" can't just mean "male." The struggle involved has cost people their lives, but the idea—the ideal—that we have inalienable rights, that we are inherently equal, that we should all have a collective say in how our societies are organized, has had a profound impact on systems of domination around the world. Hierarchies like to declare themselves the natural order, arranged by a supreme being in the office at the top. And don't even try making an appointment— He's busy into eternity. First there's God, complete with thunderbolts, guilt-inducing moral code, and penis. Then there's the king. Then the priests and the generals, usually vying for power. Beneath them are the merchant traders, beneath them the skilled craftspeople. The base of the pyramid is reserved for the laborers, usually serfs or slaves, and the base extends deep and wide. In ancient Athens, the revered origin of democracy, 90 percent of the population was enslaved. Adam Hochschild, in his extraordinary book *Bury the Chains: Prophets and Rebels in the Fight to Free an Empire's Slaves*, writes that in 1800, 80 percent of the world lived in serfdom or slavery.[99] Whatever else humanism has done, it has given people some tools to resist oppression both psychologically and politically.

So God may have given man dominion over women, animals, and the earth, but once we knock him off his throne, the question is: does the whole kingdom crumble?

Not necessarily. Putting humans at the center of the moral universe still leaves us with the dichotomy of culture vs. nature. The attributes assigned to humans are elevated into the defining distinction. Only humans are rational or self-conscious, or have agency, or are aware of our mortality, and that sets us above and apart. Humans may matter, but everything else is dead matter. Some currents of this philosophy say that humans are how the earth knows itself, the pinnacle of evolution, what the planet has done all this for. The reason to save the rainforest is not because the rainforest has the right to exist, but because there might be plants there that can cure human cancer. In this culture, humans aren't part of the natural world—we act against it and then have to weigh human "needs" against the destruction of other species. And there is nothing in humanism to argue against this behavior.

Animal Rights (AR) as a political philosophy is an offshoot of humanism. Just as the inalienable rights of liberal individualism have been extended past white rich men to include (theoretically) the rest of humanity, they should be extended to animals. Not all animals, though the Animal Rights people never come out and say that. The animals that matter are the ones that are like humans in very specific ways.

I won't eat anything that has a mother or a face. There are three unspoken characteristics that define which animals the AR people advocate for. Does it care for its young? Does it have facial features that are recognizable? Does it vocalize when it's in pain? These are characteristics that define more than who is *like us*. There are plenty of other attributes that some animals share with humans, say, hypermobile fingers or the ability to store food. But those three are the dividing lines *because they are the ones that are primary to the survival of a human child.* Without parental care, we die. The only way an infant can communicate distress—hunger, pain, fear—is by crying. And we apparently are born with a template for the human face. There is something crucial to our survival about our ability to bond mother-to-infant, an ability that depends on this recognition.[100]

And everyone who's had a baby knows about the endless hours that can slip away in simply staring into your baby's eyes. I don't even have my own and I know how compelling that experience can be. It feels primal, instinctive, I'd say "preverbal," but it doesn't lead to or need words. It doesn't feel like a stage. It feels like the thing itself, the universe entire.

These are not qualities we value for the sake of the animals. They say nothing about, for instance, an animal's ability to feel pain, or fear, or dread. Those of us who care about animal suffering are endlessly accused of sentimentality, and to our accusers the insult in that word is self-evident. The problem is that, in some sense, the accusation is true.

> For the sentimentalist it is not the object but the subject of the emotion which is important. Real love focuses on another individual: It is gladdened by his [sic] pleasure and grieved by his pain. The unreal love of the sentimentalist reaches no further than the self and gives precedence to pleasures and pains of its own, or else invents for itself a gratifying image of the pleasures and pains of its object.[101]

The quote is from Roger Scruton's *Animal Rights and Wrongs*, a book that to me was the equivalent of prodding Sappho's rubble on the beach, and yes, I am squeamish. I'm uneasy criticizing a movement that is working to stop torture. And it leaves me with a wrenching sense of moral cognitive dissonance to find my criticism expressed by someone who is otherwise repugnant to me. But sometimes your enemies are your best critics, and Scruton is precisely right about sentimentality.

The AR movement is liberal individualism applied to animals. It is a reflection of human needs and desires, not the needs and desires of animals themselves. The animals, for instance, want to hunt. They want to eat the food evolution has designed them for. Like the vegan who suggested putting a fence down the length of the Serengeti, the ARs end up having a problem with the animal nature of animals because they're arguing from a philosophical base of humanism. It's a bad idea for humans to kill other humans, for our culture to socialize its members to violence, sadism, hierarchy. We need justice, not domination, to make a human society worth the name. But those are human concepts.

To the extent that ARs stop factory farms and vivisection, on a practical level who cares about their philosophy? But if the larger goal is an egalitarian culture nestled sustainably inside its land base, the AR model will fail. It will fail because the diet the ARs aspire to is an environmental nightmare and the planet is out of topsoil. The annual grains of the vegetarians are causing mass destruction. But it will also fail because humanism contains no philosophical or moral constraints on human activity, no check on human hubris or our destructive capacity. An AR position derived from a humanist ethic will also fail because it's completely at odds with the nature of nature, including the nature of animals. Animals kill. So, for that matter, do plants. Do you know why the world smells so good after a rainstorm? The sweet scents are chemicals released by plants to attract the insects that attack their neighbors, their competitors. "Thou shalt not kill"—or the Buddhist version "Abstain from killing"— is a fine moral guideline for human society. It is nonsensical when applied to the natural world. Matthew Scully, in his book *Dominion*, uses the phrase "moral degradation" to describe cats, foxes, and weasels. "*Moral degradation*?" replies Michael Pollan in full italics.[102] Nature is no more moral than it is immoral. It's amoral, by definition. Life is literally a process of one creature eating another, whether it's bacteria breaking down plants or animals, plants strangling each other, animals going for the throat, or viruses attacking animals. "All of nature is a conjugation of the verb 'to eat,'" in the words of William Ralph Inge.

The paradigm that asks us to reject death certainly provides a simple ethical code, a code that can rally the righteous, but it is the black-and-white thinking of a child. The tremendous moral vigor that is the gift of youth seems to demand such rules, but they are essentially slogans and ethical platitudes, which are the root of fundamentalism. Adult knowledge demands more, starting with more information, and it includes the ability to incorporate that new information, to recast as necessary the behaviors informed by our values. Adults don't just absorb, they learn. The challenge of adulthood is to remember our ethical dreams and visions in the face of the complexities and frank disappointments of reality.

I used ideology like a sledgehammer and I thought I could bend the world to my demands. I couldn't. The needs of soil, the truth of the carbon cycle, and the nutritional requirements of the basic human template were a reality of brute, physical facts that would not be moved. I had built my entire identity on death being an ethical taboo, a moral horror, one that provoked a visceral shudder through body and soul. But "death-free" is not an option that the processes of life offer us. "We can dominate or we can participate, but there's no way out," a friend who grows her own food offered. We can rail and cry all we want, but in the end we have to make peace with the world, the good, green earth we claim to love so much but understand not at all. In dreams begin responsibilities, yes, but with understanding comes more. Eventually we see our only choices: the death that's destroying life or the death that's a part of life.

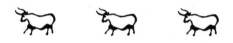

Where does that leave us morally in our dealings with each other, with animals, with the planet? First, we need to stop sentimentalizing nature. The sentimentality takes two forms. The first is the macho, Teddy Roosevelt (always elevated to his spare initials, "TR," in the pro-hunting literature) approach. Nature is violent and bloody, so there's nothing wrong with men (and it's always men who are allowed to lay claim to violence) behaving the same way. "Death by violence, death by cold, death by starvation—these are the normal endings of the stately and beautiful creatures of the wilderness. The sentimentalists who prattle about the peaceful life of nature do not realize its utter mercilessness."[103] This is observably true. If you don't know it, that's because you haven't seen enough actual nature to know how it works. It's not your fault. Even people in rural areas often live in an entirely human-made environment, buying their long-distance food from the grocery store, heating and cooling with a touch of a fossil fuel button, plugging into the TV and the internet for social contact. Rural life is urbanism with a view. The big excitement is the deer eating the shrubbery or the raccoons getting into the garbage. But the facts of nature are that the young and the old are killed. Ninety percent of most animals' babies don't make it to maturity. And as for the old, "As a rule, animals in the wild don't get good deaths surrounded by their loved ones."[104]

The TR crowd would argue that because animals do it—whatever it is, hunt, kill—humans are allowed to as well. Never mind that no (other) animal is capable of building a CAFO or keeping other animals in lifelong torment, that factory farming doesn't exist—and could never exist—in nature. The TRs have their own sentimentality and it's a maudlin attachment to their own masculinity, their own longing to invade and conquer, their own entitlement, which they project onto animals in order to claim it as the natural order. Nature is about dominance; we are but participants, they shrug.

The flip side is the ARs ignorance and denial of death, of the nature of nature. They shows their ignorance in their insistence that an agricultural diet of annual grains is sustainable and death-free, when in fact it is inherently destructive and saturated in death. This approach reaches the ridiculous with ARs trying to save animals from themselves, from their animal needs and desires, to hunt, to kill, to eat and be eaten in turn. Animal rights philosophers, writes Michael Pollan,

> show an abiding discomfort not just with our animality,
> but with the animal's animality, too. They would like nothing better than to airlift us out from nature's "intrinsic evil"
> [predation]—and then take the animals with us. You begin to wonder if their quarrel isn't really with nature itself.[105]

And the AR's denial of animals' actual nature can be stunning. I had a conversation with a vegan who had once had a small flock of chickens.

"They're the perfect animal," she gushed. Admit it, you know the tone: smug and precious and self-satisfied because her belief in nonviolence had been reaffirmed. "They don't hurt or kill anything."

They don't *what?* My mouth dropped open. It was all I could do to shut it. Chickens eat anything that moves, including insects, mice, moles, snakes, frogs, including baby chicks, including each other. I could forgive the average person who has probably never seen a real live chicken. But this was from someone who had lived with chickens. Had she really not noticed her chickens snapping at flies, ripping into mice? Was her attachment to her ideology so strong that she hadn't seen the actual facts? And not just once, but every single day?

What the ARs and the TRs have in common is this. They want to defend a political and ethical program by referring to capital-N Nature. This is a neat rhetorical trick on both sides, because who can argue with Nature? The ARs refuse the basic fact that death is the substance of life because they want to believe that they—and all humans—can eat without killing. The TRs are more realistic about life, if more repulsive. What they are missing is all the rest of nature, the part where mother bears defend their cubs with their lives; where when one goose is wounded during migration, two others go down with her to keep vigil until she recovers or dies; where plants send insecticides through their roots to ward off a companion plant's attackers; where care, compassion, and sacrifice describes the behavior of living things.

We can see whatever we want to see in "Nature." Slugs—hermaphroditic and slow-moving—make love for hours, while male dolphins kidnap and gang-rape females. Nature provides many things, but a clear-cut moral code for human concourse is not one of them.[106]

We need the moral guidance that socialization provides precisely because we are human. Our species is capable of a huge range of behaviors, from ennobling acts of courage to, yes, moral degradations like sadism and genocide. That is the particularity of our species, the joy and the horror of being human. To point to our capacity for moral agency does not require placing humans above other animals in a "natural" hierarchy, because all animals have their own specific abilities. Homing pigeons can find their way home from 1,200 miles. Whales can stay underwater for two hours. Hummingbirds process visual information so quickly that television looks like a slideshow to them. And we are not the only animal that has to teach our young. Old lobsters show their migration routes to young ones by holding claws, the way we hold hands, and walking the long miles together. A kitten without a mother to teach her may not ever learn to hunt small mammals. Such cats will let mice run all over them—though once they are shown, they never forget. A bee coming home from her first pollen run will be stroked all over by the other bees in praise and encouragement, even though she's probably carrying only one-tenth of what she will learn to in a few weeks. Beavers held in captivity without flowing water don't know how to make dams—that knowledge was passed down through the generations until humans interrupted their process of enculturation.

One day in the garden, I moved a small stone and uncovered an ant hill. The nurse ants had been using the underside of the stone as protection for the pupae until I moved it. All I had wanted was a few more inches in the lettuce bed. What resulted was panic and death. Ants running in every direction as fast as they could. No, not as fast as they could. They each grabbed a baby with their front two legs and ran with the other four, risking their own survival to save their young. I sat watching, trying not to cry. Putting the rock back would kill them. There was nothing to do but keep witness to the suffering I had brought to beings who were in the end only different from me in scale. Who among us would leave a burning building without grabbing as many infants from the daycare center as our arms could carry? And I hadn't even meant to kill ants. I'd only wanted a little more space for myself.

If you look to Nature you can find justification for almost anything. My chickens live in a hierarchy, the original pecking order. And peck they do. Some of the hens have bald patches from being incessantly plucked. This isn't about crowded conditions or an unnatural environment; they have two acres of woods and meadow and all the food they could want. This is about the nature of social animals, and there isn't any way to train them out of it. Chickens don't mourn their dead—they eat them. On slaughter day they're always underfoot, waiting for snacks. Here's how I know when there's been a hawk kill in the back meadow: I see hens with blood all down their breasts from gorging on the leftovers.

And yet, there's always more to the story. If a chicken by herself sees a predator, she'll hide as quickly and quietly as she can. But a chicken in a flock will sound the alarm, a loud, high shriek of warning. She'll draw attention to herself, put herself at risk for the good of the flock. Moral agency? What else to call it?

If you want to find blood lust you will find it. I lost thirty-nine chickens to one fox: it was carnage. A farmer down the road lost two hundred to a single coyote. Weasels, fisher cats, raccoons, all manner of creatures will kill and keep killing. But you will also find courage and sacrifice and love. Whales will carry their sick to the surface for air, and elephants *do* mourn their dead. Every year in their annual migration, when they come to the skeleton of a loved one, they'll stop and cry, cradling the skull in their trunks while they croon.

Biologist Lynn Margulis has posited that life has evolved by two species cooperating, joining together permanently to become the next level of complexity.[107] And all of those new species are in competition because they need to eat. So which do we choose to model our societies on, cooperation or competition? That's really my point: we get to choose. It's no fair falling back on Nature to justify our definingly human decisions, whether we're choosing an egalitarian culture or a hierarchical one.

Acknowledging that we get to choose, that we are political beings with big brains and no clear biological mandate beyond oxygen and food, does not put us above other life forms. We could just as easily enshrine the idea that our plasticity is a vulnerability, a human frailty, and that our capacity for hubris needs to be rigorously battled, both personally and collectively. We were not given dominion, but dependence, and only by honoring the lives that make our survival possible can our species survive. Derrick Jensen calls this the predator-prey relationship:

> When you take the life of someone to eat or otherwise use so you can survive, you become responsible for the survival and dignity of that other's community. If I eat a salmon, or rather, *when* I eat a salmon, I pledge myself to making sure that this particular run of salmon continues, and that this particular river of which the salmon are a part thrives. If I cut a tree, I make the same pledge to the larger community of which it's

a part. When I eat beef, or for that matter carrots, I pledge to eradicate factory farming.[108]

That would be a good place to start in our animist ethic. We are dependent on a million different creatures, most of them invisible to our eyes, all of them doing the work of producing or degrading that we cannot do. They are our biological forerunners, our grandparents, and without them life on this planet would cease in a matter of seconds. Between two and nine pounds of your body are bacteria, mostly in your gut helping you digest and assimilate nutrients.[109] Every one of your cells has mitochondria, with DNA separate from yours, supplying every last calorie of energy for you. Did they colonize us, domesticate us? One could argue that question. But I think the truer interpretation of these relationships is that they're symbiotic, interdependent. And an animist ethic extends way beyond dyads of mitochondria and humans, Asclepius and monarchs. An animist ethic acknowledges that every living thing is dependent on the rest, that life itself is a series of mutual dependencies. Life and death are the same moment: for someone to live, someone else does indeed have to die. To reject one is to reject the other because there is no way out. An animist ethic embraces those processes as sacred, however much our joy is mixed with pain and sorrow. Here, death is not the problem. Our commingled arrogance and ignorance are. It is our arrogance that turns death into domination, food into torture. It is our ignorance, personal and social, that stops us from facing the true cost of our dinners. And it's both that let us care only about beings that are like us, in ways that matter only to us, while discounting into extinction the lives that make ours possible.

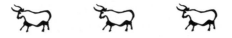

A culture worth living in would start with an attitude of reverence and awe toward this world, our home, and every last member of it. Such cultures have existed. Lisa Kemmerer explains:

The wildlife ethic of early immigrants, and the rituals and taboos surrounding that ethic such as fasting [and] prayer ... reflects an understanding of spiritual responsibility connected with the ominous task of killing kin. Behaving respectfully toward wildlife was thought *critical* to survival. Hunting, fishing, gathering, and trapping were necessary, but they were restricted and controlled by a spiritually based ethic that forbid gratuitous killing. The spiritual power of wildlife, combined with the physical dependence of human beings, colored the human-wildlife relationship. If people suffered food shortages they were not apt to say, "I cannot kill deer anymore," but rather, "Deer don't want to die for me."[110]

For some cultures, to wound an animal without killing her is so shameful that hunters will track an injured animal for days rather than return home to face approbation and scorn. The Seneca have a thanksgiving ceremony that lasts four days in which everything in their known world is named and honored.

Around the globe and across time, there are plenty of examples of cultures that approach the human project of living with humility and respect for the lives we depend on. The Chewong from Malaysia, for instance,

teach that every species inherently deserves human respect and that each possesses a unique world view. Their stories explained that the intent and behavior of any individual creature, even when it is threatening or disconcerting to humans, arises out of its unique view. This insight encouraged them to bring compassion and understanding to every encounter with other life forms.

Implicit rules that governed ethical behavior toward others arose from this core belief in the value of every species. Acceptable behavior for human beings—what was deemed good—included the need to accord respect to other species, regardless of size or appearance. Hurting or ridiculing another creature was strictly forbidden.[111]

But that attitude is only possible if we acknowledge death. This is ultimately why a vegetarian ethic will fail to produce a sustainable culture. Beyond the destructive nature of an agricultural diet, any attempt to remove ourselves emotionally, physically, spiritually from the life processes of the planet will result in a culture based on ignorance, denial, and, given our human capacity for destruction, dominance. We have to face the truth of our existence if we are to do it well. And it could be done well. We could be grateful instead of cruel, humble instead of entitled. We could accept that every living thing deserves our respect and that we are all taking turns. We could embrace our responsibility to be respectful members of this community called Earth. And only the entire culture would have to change to get us there.

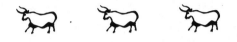

My life as a vegan was so simple. I believed that death was wrong and could be avoided by shunning animal products. My moral certainty took a number of hits over those twenty years, especially as I began to grow my own food. Ants stopped to stroke each other; spiders died for their young; butterflies taught their young the trapline of flowers from which they got nectar. Even without trying I killed them to garden. And they were like me. We shared the genes that produced our eyes and our legs, our very hearts.[112] Once I actually had my body outside and my hands in the dirt—once I could actually see insects—I could see their fear, their curiosity, their courage, their love. "Each of these tiny insects is, by definition, an animated being, a being with an anima, a soul; not a human soul indeed, but an insect soul, a thing of marvelous beauty expressing some aspect of the Divine," writes Thomas Berry.[113] I saw that. I saw it and I knew that when I killed them, I was killing someone that mattered. As a child, Abraham Lincoln stopped other children from squashing ants in the schoolyard, "contending that an ant's life was to it, as sweet as ours to us."[114] Is it a surprise that this boy grew up to sign the Emancipation Proclamation? He could include the least of us—the tiny and multilegged, the voiceless—in his circle of empathy. Varieties in human pigmentation would be nothing. Insects loved their lives: that was what I saw when I finally observed. And some of them had to die so I could live.

But just as insects—their existence, let alone their sentience—are absent from the vegetarian world view, even more so are plants. "What about plants?" was the jeer that obnoxious males would throw at me. And the problem was, I had to take it seriously. I knew other vegans who could dismiss this ethical challenge as self-evidently absurd. But how was that any different from the carnivores who dismissed my insistence that animals were sentient as self-evidently absurd? It was a question that had to be answered, and I couldn't. I would duck the issue instead, talk about grain fed to cattle instead of to hungry children. But plants were the angel I wrestled with, and I couldn't win a blessing. We think of plants "as insentient salads," in the words of Stephen Harrod Buhner.[115] I didn't want to be one of those people. But having declared death taboo and killing the consummate act of oppression, the only way out was to say that plants weren't alive, not really. Not alive like we were, us mobile animals who cared about our lives, not emotive or intelligent, not sentient. James Lovelock writes:

> Mammals first, of course, for toads and frogs seem less alive, and trees and plants less still, and lichens, algae, and soil bacteria, hardly alive at all. Much of the instinctive objection to viewing the Earth as a living system comes from our zoocentrism, the tendency to consider ourselves, and animals, as more alive than other living organisms.[116]

I couldn't prove that plants weren't sentient. But more importantly, I didn't *want* to prove it. I wanted to believe in what Joanne Elizabeth Lauck calls "the perennial wisdom of indigenous cultures that believed we were never alone—that we were immersed in a sentient world."[117]

If they were sentient, I couldn't kill them. So I had to make another category in my head: alive and honored, respected and thanked, but not really sentient. The more I interacted with plants—the more I took joy in their tiny, tender radicles, listened to their song of color and scent, watched them struggle and reach and climb, learned their language—the less that category made any sense. What right did I have to plant tomatoes, knowing they'd be dead from frost by the end of September? They can live ten years in the tropics, their native home. What right did I have to subjugate them to my needs, my will? At least animals could try to get away. Plants were stuck wherever I put them and couldn't fight back as I hacked off chunks of their bodies, stole their babies.

And then I would retreat, intellectually, emotionally, because I had to eat something and vegan was righteous, wasn't it? Vegan was just, sustainable, life-affirming. All the books—and all my friends—said so. I'd long ago crossed the line into radical, political, uncompromising. Wasn't questioning the tenets of veganism automatically conservative, anti-animal, on the side of loggers and rapists and every Big Bad Evil Thing I had to stop?

But, as I was forced to acknowledge, I had to eat. So I grew my food and loved my plants and said I was sorry when harvest came and hoped it was enough. And I also gathered more information, the beginning place of knowledge. Plants breathe in CO2, and during photosynthesis they break apart the carbon and the oxygen, keeping the carbon to build and fuel their bodies and releasing the oxygen. Over 500 million years, plant sequestration of carbon let the atmospheric oxygen levels rise to 21 percent, enough for the rest of us to come into being.

In *The Lost Language of Plants*, Stephen Harrod Buhner presents page after page detailing what plants do. They defend themselves. They protect each other. They communicate. They call out to other plant species, asking them to join in forming a resilient community. They sometimes sacrifice themselves for the good of all. They respond. They talk. They have meaning and they make meaning. They are capable of agency and courage and self-awareness. They make life possible. Any human who either breathes oxygen or eats food should read his book.

Where we use locomotion and opposable thumbs, plants use chemicals. That is the difference between us. Plants produce

> hundreds of thousands, perhaps millions of complex, second-ary compounds ... Adding to the complexity, all these compounds can be made using different metabolic pathways—different construction techniques, as it were—and each family of secondary metabolites can contain incredible numbers of substances. Simply altering the relationship between four sugar molecules, for instance, can create more than 35,000 different compounds. More than 10,000 alkaloids, 20,000 terpenes, and 8000 polyphenols are known ... Through complex feedback loops, plants constantly sense what is happening in the world around them and, in response, vary the numbers, combinations, and amounts of the phytochemicals they make.[118]

These chemicals are used for obvious tasks like fighting off insects, fungi, or bacteria. Susan Allport dubs phyto-chemicals "plants' armed services. Plants cannot flee from hungry predators, of course, so they became experts in chemical warfare instead."[119] They also use chemicals to call pollinators and protectors with a specificity that is exquisite enough to stop your breath. Saguaro cacti need a unique species of *Drosophila* fly. The cacti release a volatile steroidal compound that the flies must have to reach sexual maturity and reproduce. In return, the flies and their larva eat the decaying parts of the cacti, keeping the plants healthy. The volatiles are so precise that for 6,803 larvae on the average saguaro cactus, only one is not the correct species.[120] Each of the world's seven hundred plus species of figs has its own specific fig wasp, wasps who hand pollinate that fig's seeds. In some forests, 70 percent of vertebrate diets are composed of these figs.[121]

And it's not just insects who respond to these chemical cues. Most of these chemicals have no scent, but are instead received by receptors called vomeronasal organs (VNOs) which all vertebrates have. The only function that VNOs perform is to attach to the minute amounts of aromatic chemicals that plants and animals give off and transport them to the brain. VNOs are how bees are able to locate and then remember the exact location of all the flowering plants within a sixty mile radius. It's because of VNOs that women living together will synchronize menstrual cycles.

Plants are in constant communication with each other. "Each plant, plant neighborhood, plant community, ecosystem, and biome has messages flowing through it constantly—trillions and trillions of messages at the same time."[122] Any place that roots touch other roots or their shared mycelial network, they can also exchange chemistries, medicines. One plant will send out a chemical distress call. The others respond with precise antibiotics, antifungals, antimicrobials, or pesticides to help. Like my chickens when they sight a hawk, plants will give out an alarm call when a predator is near. Lima beans will release chemicals that warn other lima beans when they are being attacked by spider mites.[123] When something ambulatory brushes past a plant in the woods, not only does the affected plant respond by stiffening as best it can, it also sends out a chemical warning that allows all the plants nearby to stiffen their branches in preparation.

And there's more. Buhner talks about archipelagoes of plant communities, groupings of intercommunicating plants around a dominant or keystone species, usually a tree. These archipelagoes form in response to mysterious and unpredictable cues, and often announce the wholesale movement of ecosystems. The process begins with an outrider or pioneer plant, who literally prepares the soil for its cohorts. When the soil is ready, the nurse plant sends out the chemical message: *join me*. What happens next is astounding.

> Though wind, ants, and burrowing animals may sometimes disperse keystone seeds to the new locations, researchers have found that mere wind and animal dispersal patterns cannot explain how the seeds move. The distances are too far, the dispersal patterns too unusual. But by whatever means, the seeds answer the chemical call sent by the nurse plants.[124]

Once established, the keystone plant then calls the bacteria, mycelia, plants, insects, and other animals necessary to build a healthy and resilient community. The keystone's chemistries arrange the other species and direct their behavior. "This capacity of keystone species to 'teach' their plant communities how to act was widely recognized in indigenous and folk taxonomies."[125] Elder trees are called *elders* for a reason.

> Among many indigenous and folk people it is said that the elder tree 'teaches the plants what to do and how to grow,' and that without its presence the local plant community will become confused ... Other indigenous peoples, recognizing the nature and function of keystone species, have said that 'the trees are the teachers of the law.'"[126]

The individual plants will not achieve the same growth when in a relationship with a keystone species, but together "they create *more* biomass than if grown separately, even if supplied with all the water and nutrients they need."[127] They use more CO_2, grow denser root systems, create more extensive canopies and hence more photosynthesis, store more water both internally and in the soil, and attract a wider range of soil organisms. Concludes Buhner, "A plant community is far more than the sum of its parts."[128]

Not only do trees create rain. They typically use only one-third of the water they lift from the soil for themselves. The other two-thirds are for the tree's cohorts.[129] And it goes beyond water. "Plants *always* produce more chemistries than they need for their own health: these chemicals are released into plant communities and ecosystems to maintain them."[130] Plant chemistries, air- or soil-borne, affect seed germination, mitochondrial oxygen usage, bacterial respiration and hence growth, plant respiration, and humic acid formation. They literally control life on earth.

Plants may not respond in a way that is obvious to our ambulating species, but they do respond. It's only that they are moving at a speed that we have to work to understand. Start with the fact that plants can live thousands of years. There's a 43,000 year old holly in

Tasmania, a creosote that is 18,000 years old, a grass colony that's 1,000.[131] This is almost inconceivable to our human timescale. Writes Buhner,

> plants and plant communities possess tremendous powers of movement... their movement shows intention... they can cross thousands of miles when motivated and ... their movement patterns are not random but are determined by large-scale feedback loops millions of years old. On a short, localized scale: Climbing plants that need support will grow toward a trellis, and if the trellis is shifted the plants will change direction. On long scales this can be even more pronounced, though it is harder to see... Plants circulate throughout ecosystems, between ecosystems and across and between continents; the longest seed dispersal distance known (without human help) is 15,000 miles. Plants, in fact, move themselves throughout land masses and across distances that mere seed dispersal dynamics and mathematics cannot explain. The places they move to and the ways that they arrange themselves in ecosystems are not accidental and are not random.[132]

At what point are you, vegetarian or carnivore, willing to acknowledge that plants are sentient? When you find out that a girdled tree will die on its own, but will survive many years if surrounded by its chosen community? Other plants will send an injured one "carbon, phosphorus, sugars and more."[133] How is this different from whales carrying their sick loved ones to the surface? Why don't we want to include plants in the circle of us? We share 50 percent of our DNA.

Or think about the behavior of spruces when under attack by spruce budworms. Most of the trees produce terpenes that kill the budworms, but a few trees don't. These trees are not sick or defective. Scientists have discovered that the trees are just as capable of producing the necessary defenses. They are choosing not to. Why? "By not raising antifeedant actions in all the trees, the forest makes sure that resistance is not developed in spruce budworms as it does in crop insects exposed to pesticides. Plant communities literally set aside plants for the insects to consume so as not to force genetic rearrangement and the development of resistance."[134] How else to describe this behavior (can you agree that this is *behavior*, not phenomenon?) without acknowledging that these trees are willfully sacrificing themselves for the good of their community?

The understanding of almost all nonindustrial cultures is that "humans are the offspring of the plants."[135] Some cultures consider trees our parents. From an evolutionary perspective, that is a simple truth, but it's one that this culture, including the subculture of vegetarians, does its best to forget, even when science backs it up. But there are those of us who still remember:

> Among widely diverse nonindustrial cultures the members whose specialty was plant medicines, *vegetalistas*, described their experiences remarkably similarly *irrespective of culture, continents, or time*. The vast majority ... told interviewers that they did not obtain their knowledge of plant medicines from the exercise of reason or through trial and error. They were uniformly consistent in saying that their personal and cultural knowledge of the additional actions of plants came from "nonordinary" experiences, specifically: dreams, visions, direct communications from the plant, or sacred beings.[136]

There is a profound moment where science and ancient wisdom sometimes meet. Nobel Laureate Barbara McClintock, who studied corn genetics, has said it was the corn that told her what she needed to know. All it asked for in return was care and respect.[137] "Corn is our Parent and Elder," explains Patrisia Gonzales Patzin. "Many traditional people speak of corn as a living being, each one unique like a human being."[138] Meanwhile the Winnebago believe that "when gathering plants as medicine, if you tell them what you need them to do and ask them to put forth their strength on your behalf they will do so."[139] The Iroquois are taught to pray to medicinal plants for help. They believe that the plant will tell other plants, who will respond by offering more healing power. The Cherokee and Creek say that because we are the children of plants, they will take pity on us and help us. "There is deep wisdom in this," writes Buhner.

> Understanding ourselves to be the offspring, the children, of the plants naturally engenders a familial bond. It shifts the focus of our relationship from one of plants as resources to them being senior, caring members of the same family. More than that, the power lies with the plants, not with us. *We* are *their* children; they are not our property.[140]

This is the knowledge—the wisdom—that we will have to remember if we are to have any hope of creating a sustainable culture. The mechanistic model of the earth as "a ball of resources inhabited by human beings hurtling through space"[141] has produced a planet of dead zones, deserts, and missing species—our parents, our siblings. The moral vegetarians have proven themselves willing to take ethical risks and to make personal sacrifices. They have a deep and abiding passion for justice, for animals, for the planet. I know how deep and how abiding, because the same passion runs in me as strong and instinctive as salmon seeking home. I am not questioning vegetarian commitment or integrity. But the vegetarian ethic is still ultimately a variation on the mechanistic model. It simply extends our morality, whether humanist or religious, to a few animals that are similar to us. The rest of the world—the living, sentient, communicating agents who make oxygen and soil, rain and biomass—those billions of creatures don't count. They make life and they are life, but the vegetarian ethic declares them, and thus the world entire, dead matter. Despite the vegetarians' unassailable longings to create a culture verdant with justice and compassion, their ethic is still part of the paradigm that's destroying the world.

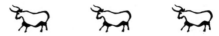

Where was I going to draw the line? That was the question, my personal, political, spiritual agony. Mammals, fish, insects, plants, plankton, bacteria? Was the least of us going to be an "us"? And if "what" became "who," then what would be left to eat?

I have my answer, finally. I'm not going to draw a line. I'm going to draw a circle.

It's so simple, as simple, really, as my vegan morality: we need to be a part of the world to know it. And when we join, when we participate, we see that life and death can't be separated any more than night and day. I will face what is dying to feed me and I will do my best to ensure it is individuals—cared for, respected—not entire species; that soil—the work of our grandparents for half a billion years— is built, not destroyed; that the rivers keep their waters and their wetlands and that the oil stays in the ground. Only then can I claim the title "adult." The circle becomes a spiral, moving across space and time, our other partners in this cosmic project. But even a spiral is too singular, and life—its creation, its sustenance—is vastly, profoundly more complex than what the human brain could ever comprehend. So the spiral has to branch, branch again, into fractals of contact, communication, response, until it's a web. But a web is still static, and life changes. Each individual life, precious to its bearer, will begin and end, just as each species, each mountain, each star, will die. In the end, that line is not a web either, it's a flow, a living river, and we are the boatmen alighting on its surface, waiting for the fish to eat us, to take us home.

CHAPTER 3
Political Vegetarians

Start with a cow, an animal who has evolved to do one thing exquisitely: take cellulose—ubiquitous, non-nutritious grass—and turn it into mass and motion. Like all members of a healthy biotic community, our cow is producing food for someone else. Her manure feeds soil, plants, insects; the mechanical action of her teeth and her hooves help the grasslands stay diverse; her digestive processes free up nutrients, and not just for her, but for the whole community; and her body will become a meal for predators, scavengers, and degraders of all sizes. She has help, too, like we all do: friendly bacteria fill her rumen to do the actual work of breaking down that cellulose. She gives them a home and then she eats them. And it's more than just bacteria she's nurturing. There are fungi, yeast, and protozoans. Every gallon (and she's got between twenty-five and thirty) of rumen capacity can contain "200 trillion bacteria and 4 billion protozoans" with fungi and yeast by the millions.[1] Has she domesticated them, or have they colonized her? This is the only question that can arise from an epistemology of domination, a culture saturated in power and hierarchy and its defenders. But life is ultimately a cooperative process, unitary in its goal: more life. Observing our cow—observing across the long arc of evolution—can reveal both the complex dependencies of living communities and where human culture has gone so dreadfully wrong.

All animals have evolved in an environment dense with microbes. Just as plants do the work of producing, bacteria do most of the work of degrading, and those activities, producing and degrading, are the only two functions necessary for life. What animals have done is figure out how to work with and around bacteria. We developed digestive tracts in which we could carry the helpful ones around with us. Explains Roderick I. Mackie:

> Large populations of microorganisms inhabit the gastrointestinal tract of all animals and form a closely integrated ecological unit with the host. This complex mixed, microbial culture comprising bacteria, ciliate and flagellate protozoa, anaerobic phycomycete fungi as well as bacteriophage can be considered as the most metabolically adaptable and rapidly renewable organ of the body which plays a vital role in the normal nutritional, physiological, immunological and protective functions of the host animal.[2]

You could also look at this from the bacteria's perspective: they discovered how to get locomoted, fed, and protected by helping animals survive. Of course, bacteria might also want to eat their host, or they might want to eat their host's food. So animals have found three ways to handle that potential conflict.

The first is the competition model used by carnivores. The animal's immune system keeps the microbes in the digestive tract from eating the animal. Antimicrobial acid is secreted by the animal's stomach, which prevents the bacteria from eating the carnivore's food. The host then uses digestive enzymes to further break down food. This process means quick transit through the stomach, accompanied by a slower rate of passage through the lower digestive tract, where the food—now "enzymic digestive products"—is absorbed. It means a larger number of microbes in the hind gut, as opposed to the stomach. And I'm sorry, vegetarians, but this exactly describes the human digestive system, especially in contrast with herbivores.

The cooperation model lets animals utilize the abundant cellulose of the plant world. Fifty percent of the carbon on our planet is cellulose.[3] The carbohydrate polymers that make up plant cell walls are indigestible to most animals and all mammals. Cellulose can only be broken down by microbial fermentation. The whole point of the ruminant's digestion is to keep food in the vast fermentative vat of its rumen so the bacteria have time to digest the cellulose. A cow regurgitates and rechews her food 500 times a day, for eight hours, approximating 25,000 chews.[4] A cow is sacrificing the dietary protein in the grass, letting the microbes eat it instead. In the end, however, she trades in that poor quality plant protein for good quality microbial protein. This is what's happening inside a cow: she feeds grass to the bacteria, and then she eats them.[5]

The third model is the combined competition-cooperation model. This method is used by "horses, elephants, hyraxes, rodents, and lagomorphs (hares and rabbits) but is probably best exemplified in the termites."[6] The host animal has enzymes that break down what is ingested, and the resulting enzymic products are absorbed *before* microbial fermentation. This is very clever because

> the host obtains not only the nutrients digested by its own enzymes but also fermentation products from materials its enzymes cannot digest ... A disadvantage of the combination model is that, although the host absorbs the fermentation end-products, the microbial cells themselves cannot be used as a nutrient source. Some animals have overcome this deficiency by consuming the faeces or cecal content containing the microbes using a strategy termed coprophagy or cecotrophy respectively.[7]

Yum.

All three of the strategies are elegant ways of recycling the sun's energy, the true power source of life. Can't photosynthesize? Eat someone who can. Can't digest their cellulose body? Eat someone who can. Rodney Heitschmidt and Jerry Stuth point out that "[h]umankind has historically fostered and relied upon livestock grazing for a substantial portion of its livelihood because it is the only process capable of converting the energy in grassland vegetation into an energy source directly consumable by humans."[8] Nineteen billion metric tons of vegetation are produced by plants in grasslands and savannas, and we can't eat them. [9] Humans and ruminants are not naturally in competition for the same meal: this is where the political vegetarians have gone wrong. Yes, industrial culture has been stuffing grain into as many animals as it can. But it's the logic of industrial capitalism that's dictating that diet, not nature.

What happens when you take our cow, an animal filled with friendly bacteria hungry for cellulose, and feed her grain? Carnivore stomachs like ours are acidic to kill bacteria competing for our food. The cow's rumen, however, is neutral, because she's *encouraging* bacteria, bacteria she depends on. But grain turns her normally neutral rumen acid, which makes her sick. Bloat, for instance, is caused by grain feeding. Rumination slows to a halt, and a "layer of foam slime" traps the gas that is a natural byproduct of fermentation.[10] The rumen swells until it suffocates the animal. Then there's acidosis. This disease causes animals to "go off their feed, pant and salivate excessively, paw and scratch their bellies, and eat dirt."[11] Acidosis can lead to "diarrhea, ulcers, bloat, pneumonitis, liver disease ... the full panoply of feedlot diseases—pneumonia, coccidiosis, enterotoxemia, feedlot polio."[12] The acid eats through the rumen, letting bacteria into the cow's bloodstream. Since the liver's function is to clean the blood, the microbes end up in the cow's liver, causing abscesses. Somewhere between 15 and 38 percent of beef cattle have abscessed livers at death.[13] Michael Pollan sums up, "Much like modern humans, modern cattle are susceptible to a set of relatively new diseases of civilization."[14]

E. Coli, for example, is one of the premier diseases of civilization, in this case the end point of industrial agriculture. *Escherichia coli* is a common resident in both humans and cows. Some variants are harmless; others are even useful to us. But E. Coli 0157:H7 causes intestinal bleeding that can result in kidney failure, brain damage, and death. The harmless strains of E. Coli die out in the unnaturally acidic digestive tract of unnaturally fed cattle. But E. Coli 0157: H7 can survive a highly acidic environment. In other words, all that's left is the bacteria that can kill us.

Researchers from Cornell showed that E. Coli 0157:H7 could be stopped by a very simple action: feeding cows hay for the last five days of their lives.[15] But the economic insanity that has created corn-fed cattle can't see reason. It can only see the mountain of corn, cheaper to buy than it is to grow, subsidized by thousands of years of natural capital—prairie topsoil, fossil fuel, aquifer water—and the US taxpayer.

My first argument against the political vegetarians isn't an argument at all: it's an agreement. Factory farming is a nightmare, from every angle: ethically, ecologically, nutritionally. There's no word besides torture to describe the experience of laying hens in battery cages, so crowded they can't lie down or open their wings, driven insane by the bright glare of lights that stay on forever. Torture also describes what happens to pigs, animals that are smarter than dogs, so smart in fact that if they had digits instead of hooves they could probably learn some rudimentary sign language:

> The air in hog factories is laden with dust, dander, and noxious gases, which are produced as the animals' urine and feces build up inside the sheds ... [R]espiratory disease is rampant.... [T]he sows are confined in gestation crates — small metal pens just two feet wide that prevent sows from turning around or even lying down comfortably... With barely enough room to stand up and lie down and no straw or other type of bedding to speak of, many suffer from sores on their shoulders and knees.... The unnatural flooring and lack of exercise causes obesity and crippling leg disorders, while the deprived environment produces neurotic coping behaviors such as repetitive bar biting and sham chewing (chewing nothing)....
> [T]hey are forced to live in their own feces, urine, vomit and even amid the corpses of other pigs.[16]

This tortuous life ends at the slaughterhouse, where, if not properly stunned and killed, they may be boiled alive in a rendering vat. No moral person can face these facts without a sickening of the spirit. Where I part company with the political vegetarians is when they conflate factory farming with any and all meat. "So you're an environ-mentalist? Why are you still eating meat?" trumpeted Jim Motavalli of *E Magazine* in an article that got posted on just about every listserv I was on. If the title had put "factory-farmed" in front of "meat" it would be substantially more accurate. Some of what's in that article would even be true. But most political vegetarians refuse to acknowl-edge the distinction. Part of this is simply ignorance: they don't know that cows eat grass anymore than they know that soil eats cows. But some of it is emotional dishonesty. These vegetarians aren't looking for truths about sustainability or justice. They're looking for the small slice of facts that will shore up their ideology, their identities. This is where politics becomes religion, psychologically speaking, where the seeker is looking for reaffirmation of her beliefs rather than active knowledge of the world. I was one such believer; the above could be written in a very personal first person rather than the distancing third. What cracked my beliefs open wasn't the facts about agriculture, the death and destruction it entails. What wore through the fabric of my faith was illness and exhaustion. Only then was I willing to turn and face whole sections of knowledge. I had gathered and then abandoned them, and they stood waiting like hungry children with the demands that chil-dren are entitled to make on adults. Knowledge makes similar claims on our attention, on our hearts, on our actions. Knowledge about factory farming led me to veganism: it required action. Most vegetar-ians have experienced the same vocation: called by justice to right the world. What I am asking is for you to hear that call again.

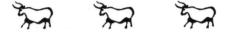

"The 4.8 pounds of grain fed to cattle to produce one pound of beef for human beings represents a colossal waste of resources in a world still teeming with people who suffer from profound hunger and malnutrition," writes Jim Motavalli.[17] Yes, it is a waste, but not for the reasons he thinks. As we have seen in abundance, growing that grain will require the felling of forests, the plowing of prairies, the draining of wetlands, and the destruction of topsoil. In most places on earth, it will never be sustainable, and where it just possibly might be, it will require rotation with animals on pasture. And it's ridiculous to the point of insanity to take that world-destroying grain and feed it to a ruminant who could have happily subsisted on those now extinct forests, grasslands, and wetlands of our planet, while *building* topsoil and species diversity.

So you're an environmentalist; why are you still eating annual monocrops?

"According to the British group Vegfam, a 10-acre farm can support 60 people growing soybeans, 24 people growing wheat, 10 people growing corn and only two producing cattle," Motavalli continues. And he believes them? Set aside the fact that a diet of soy, wheat, or corn will result in massive malnutrition—along with fun stuff like kwashiorkor, pellagra, retardation, blindness—and ultimately death. The figure of two cattle might be true if you assume grain feeding, though I can't make the math come out. By contrast, a ten acre farm of perennial polyculture in a mid-Atlantic climate could produce:

3,000 eggs
1,000 broilers
80 stewing hens
2,000 pounds of beef
2,500 pounds of pork
100 turkeys
50 rabbits

Not to mention a few inches of topsoil.[18] This is the amount of food that Joel Salatin—one of the high priests of the local, sustainable movement—produces on ten acres of his Polyface Farm in Virginia. The chickens get some supplemental grain; everything else eats grass. That's 6,800,050 calories.[19] Figuring 720,000 calories a year (2,000 x 365) per person, if they eat *nothing* but the above, that's enough to support at least nine people and support them in full health by providing essential protein and fat. Add in the organ meats and the vast quantities of nutritious bone broth that could be prepared, and you have more crucial animal fats and fat-soluble vitamins.

As I have said, two-thirds of the world is utterly unsuited to growing grain. And not just mountain tops in far distant Nepal, but right here in, say, New England. Cows are what grow here. So are deer, in their forest-destroying abundance. To eat the supposedly earth-friendly diet Motavalli is suggesting means that everyone in a cold, hot, wet, or dry climate would have to be dependent on the American Midwest, with its devastated prairies and ghostly Limberlost, and its ever shrinking soil, rivers, and aquifers. It also means dependence on coal or oil to ship that grain two thousand miles. So you're an environmentalist; why are you still eating outside your bioregion?

"A pound of wheat can be grown with 60 pounds of water, whereas a pound of meat requires 2,500 to 6,000 pounds."[20] One more time: only if you're feeding them grain. On pasture, beef cattle will drink eight to fifteen gallons of water a day. The average pasture-raised steer takes 21 months to reach market weight.[21] That's 630 days, at eight pounds a gallon, for a total of anywhere between 40,320-75,600 pounds of water total *for an entire cow*. That's 450-500 pound of meat, with another 146 pounds of fat and bone trimmed off, which in an earlier, saner era would have been valued for food as well. Taking the mean of 475 pounds, the midpoint of 57,960 gallons yields a figure of 122 pounds of water per pound of meat, not Motavalli's 2,500 to 6,000, a much more appropriate use of resources and a more accurate fact. And I'm only figuring for the muscle meat, not the organ meats, which are the most nutritionally dense and historically valued parts of the animal.

A dairy cow will drink more water, anywhere from twenty-five to fifty gallons, depending on the breed, the temperature, and how many gallons of milk she's producing. For nine gallons of milk, she drinks about eighteen gallons of water, a roughly two-to-one ratio. Never mind water into wine: this is the original life-affirming transmutation.

More importantly, compare the nutrition in that pound of wheat against that pound of beef. The beef contains almost twice as many calories (592 vs. 339, per 100 grams). Calories are simply energy, which means the beef is providing substantially more. If you want to compare pounds of water for calories (energy) produced, wheat and grass-fed beef end up almost even. For wheat, sixty pounds of water produces 1524.45 calories, or 25.7 calories per pound of water. For grass-fed beef, it's twenty-two calories from a pound of water.

And there's more than simple energy: those beef calories contain more nutrients, especially essential protein and fat. The numbers on those are 21 g vs. 13.7 g, and 8.55 vs. 1.87 g, respectively.[22] It's also crucial to understand that the protein in the beef contains the full spectrum of necessary amino acids and is easy for humans to assimilate, while the protein in the wheat is both low-quality and largely inaccessible because it comes wrapped in indigestible cellulose. For the water used, beef is better.

More importantly, cows are not the most water-efficient ruminants. They're inappropriate for many arid environments, particularly landscapes where they didn't evolve. Their hooves and teeth are too destructive to the native plants and they simply drink too much. An antelope, a buffalo, a bighorn sheep, a zebra, or a camel would be better suited to those biotic communities—and the water per calorie and water per nutrient ratio would further outstrip wheat.

But most importantly, animals aren't ever-expanding water balloons. For a steer, almost all of that water will be returned in the form of urine and feces laden with nutrients and bacteria, value-added as it were, to the land that needs it. For a dairy animal, there's also milk. In an area like Massachusetts—cold, rocky, steep, with forty-three inches of rainfall a year—dairy makes sense. That's why if I say "Vermont" you're likely to picture a cow. Or you might cut right to the chase and picture Ben and Jerry. In a dry area like New Mexico, dairy makes a lot less sense. And plowing up that New Mexico land for annual grains makes even less. Attempting annual crops will destroy that land forever. That is the point the political vegetarians need to understand. In the end all our calculations don't matter. Who cares if more food can be produced by farming when farming is destroying the world?

The logic of the land tells us to eat the animals that can eat the tough cellulose that survives there. But the logic of the vegans leads us away from the local, our only chance of being sustainable, back to the desperate Mississippi and her dying wetlands, her eroding delta. Yes, eating grain directly is less water-intensive than eating grain-fed beef. But why eat either? Animals integrated into appropriate polycultures destroy nothing.

So you're an environmentalist; why are you killing a distant river with every bite?

"Energy-intensive US factory farms generated 1.4 billion tons of animal waste in 1996, which ... pollutes American waterways more than all other industrial sources combined."[23] Yes, because cattle are standing around in giant feedlots ingesting corn rather than grazing on grass, where they belong. Manure is a biological gift, not a waste. It only became a waste when the annual monocrops, especially corn, pushed out the grasslands, and cattle were shifted to CAFOs. Factory farms are energy intensive because the animals are being raised in a way that goes against nature, and it takes energy to fight nature. The cycles—the hydrological cycle, the mineral cycle with its nesting nitrogen, carbon, and calcium cycles—have been disrupted by the human activity of agriculture, an activity more like war than anything else.

Up until about 1950, agriculture was still limited by the amount of energy that fell from the sun. What that meant practically was that animals had to be integrated into small farms because their manure— the best source of naturally occurring nitrogen—was needed there. Animals ate the cellulose in pastures, pastures rotated with annual crops. In most places, the soil wore out and eventually imperialism was the final result, but there were limits of biology and physics— building blocks and energy. Nitrogen was prized, and every molecule of that was used by hungry plants and ultimately hungry humans. This is the chemistry we should learn like a liturgy: life is spoken in the language of nitrogen. You've probably heard that amino acids are the building blocks of protein. Well, nitrogen is the building block of amino acids, the alphabet of DNA.

While nitrogen is abundant in the atmosphere, it's not available for life processes since it's paired in tight bonds. To be available, those pairs must be split and then rejoined to hydrogen atoms. This is called "fixing" nitrogen. If you're a gardener, you've probably read that leguminous plants "fix" nitrogen. As usual it's the bacteria doing the work, but these particular bacteria live in a symbiotic relationship with leguminous plants, trading in the nitrogen for a droplet of plant sugar. This is where essentially all the fixed nitrogen on the earth started.[24] A hundred years ago, European scientists realized that nitrogen was essentially a limiting factor for humanity, and that limit would bring certain starvation. Asian agronomists came to much the same conclusion half a century later, and that may well have played a part in China's diplomatic overtures to the US. The first large purchase Beijing made after Nixon's historic visit was of gigantic factories to produce nitrogen fertilizer.[25]

Those massive fertilizer factories depend on two things: fossil fuel and a man named Fritz Haber. The Haber-Bosch process uses tremendous heat and pressure to force nitrogen and hydrogen together. This creates a usable form of nitrogen. Large quantities of electricity are necessary to produce the heat and pressure, and large quantities of coal, oil, or gas are necessary to produce the hydrogen. It relies on fossil fuel from beginning to end.

Understand the profound impact the Haber-Bosch process has had on the planet: two out of five people are only alive because of it.[26] And, instead of running on the sun, modern agriculture runs on fossil fuel. Unhooked from the limits of a biological system, an industrial system sprang to life in 1947, when a munitions plant in Alabama retooled itself for chemical fertilizer. A munitions plant? Surely you realize by now that my agriculture-as-war construction is no metaphor.

Remember that annual plants only get their day in the sun after a catastrophe opens a niche in a perennial polyculture. Writes Richard Manning:

> Farming is the process of ripping that niche open again and again. It is an annual artificial catastrophe, and it requires the equivalent of three or four tons of TNT per acre for a modern American farm. Iowa's fields require the energy of 4,000 Nagasaki bombs every year.[27]

Haber discovered his process during Germany's First World War effort. Nitrogen makes great bombs. Germany's nitrates came from guano in Chilean mines, until Britain disrupted the German supply. Haber's discovery kept Germany in the war business. It also won him

a Nobel Prize. Haber also developed poison gases, including am-
monia, chlorine, and the Holocaust horror of Zyklon B. He oversaw
the first gas attack ever on April 22, 1915.[28] This overlap between
war and agriculture will only surprise you if you believe the myth of
civilization or the myth of the political vegetarians, which end up
substantially the same since their genesis is the same: agriculture and
its annual monocrops. The myth is that civilization is progress, for
human rights, human health, and human culture. The myth continues: agriculture's foods are the foods of peace and justice. A poster
entitled "How To Build Global Community" lists activities like "Look
for fair trade and union labels," "Question consumption," and "Hon-
or everyone's holidays." And then, "Enjoy vegetables, beans and grains
in your diet." And if those things don't grow where I live? How does
my consumption of strawberries from Chile, snap peas from China,
or corn from Iowa build anything but more exploitation and destruction? What if I want to preserve, say, biodiversity, rivers, topsoil, self-
sufficient human communities around the globe? What that poster
should say is "Know your land and your water, your local farmers
and their animals. Eat what grows sustainably in your foodshed,"
followed by "Get a vasectomy." But plowshares and swords are both
the weapons of the civilized. Swords take the land that the plowshares
will destroy, requiring more swords. And the blood of the indigenous
makes a good fertilizer for a season or two.

Since 1947, the fertilizer has come from fossil fuel. That was
about the point when the world's arable soil was almost out of fertility, agriculture having run its totalizing trajectory. Instead of a biologic
correction against a species on overshoot, what happened instead was
the green revolution. Richard Manning puts it well: "With the possible exception of the domestication of wheat, the green revolution is
the worst thing that has ever happened to the planet."[29]

Breaking our dependence on the sun and nature's fertility meant
an explosion in grain production and a concomitant expansion in
the human population. There are now over 6 billion humans. Understand: billions of us are only here because of fossil fuel, because we
figured out how to transform stored energy into edible energy. There
is nowhere else to get that energy. As the natural gas and oil get more

expensive, and then prohibitively expensive, there will be no way to keep that grain coming. And then? It doesn't sound like a party I want to attend.

But it's the industrialization of agriculture that has made factory farming possible. This is another point that political vegetarians need to understand. Animals were taken off their native food, out of their natural life patterns, because they weren't needed on farms anymore. Their ability to turn cellulose into protein wasn't an asset when corn could be grown so densely, so cheaply out of bare land and fossil fuel. And then the truly bizarre began to make economic sense: the mountain of corn that the US produced had nowhere else to go but into animals. Cheap corn, as George Pyle says, "has encouraged the creation of a factory farm system for beef, pigs and poultry that would ... not exist otherwise."[30] Or as Michael Pollan puts it, "The urbanization of America's animal population would never have taken place if not for the advent of cheap, federally subsidized corn."[31]

Between 1963 and 1997, worldwide crop yields doubled. This doubling came at a cost: fertilizer use increased by 645 percent between 1961 and 1996.[32] George Pyle writes, "The practice of repeatedly plowing the fields, removing the covering of grasses, and poisoning the bugs and the weeds robs the soil of most of its life-giving characteristics. Because this deep-seated soil cannot trap nitrogen the way living soil can, the farmer needs to pour on chemical fertilizers."[33] We've already seen how these crops demand more water from dying rivers, sinking water tables, emptied aquifers, how irrigation creates a wasteland of salt-caked desert. My point here is that this abundance of grain is no true abundance. When the vegetarians claim, for instance, that "Britain could support a population of 250 million on an all-vegetable diet"[34] they are basing those numbers on the overinflated production only made possible by fertilizer from fossil fuel. Set aside the soil loss, the salinization, the emptied rivers. Whether fed to people or animals, the grain in those numbers is essentially fossil fuel on a stalk.

"Ever since we ran out of arable land, food is oil," writes Richard Manning.[35] A typical farm in 1940 "produced two calories of food energy for every calorie of fossil energy used. By 1974 ... that ratio was

1:1." As of now, it takes *more* than a calorie of fossil fuel to produce a calorie of food energy for humans—somewhere between four and ten calories of fossil fuel for a calorie of food.[36] The fossil fuel is in both the fertilizer and the pesticides, and it's essential to the machinery needed to plant, harvest, process, and transport grain. All told, an acre of corn drinks about fifty gallons of oil.[37]

The political vegetarians, however noble their intentions, are planning a planetary diet in complete ignorance of where food comes from. Advocates like Peter Singer and John Robbins want us to grow annual grains and no animals at all. Set aside the topsoil, water, climate, and topography problems. What is going to fertilize that grain? Peter, John: *what is going to feed your food?* Vegetarians, like everyone else in an urban industrial culture, have no concept that plants need to eat, that soil is alive and hungry. They seem shocked when I ask them what will feed their food. Do plants *eat?* their expressions say. They don't just ... happen? There was a time when I didn't know either, so I'm patient. But eventually the question has to be answered: fossil fuel or manure?

And when we're tired of the acid rain and the oil slicks, the melting glaciers and the asthma? And when the oil starts to run low? What if we want to boycott corrupt monarchies or imperialist wars? These are the weft of an oil economy, and ecological devastation is the warp. Or what if we're uneasy about our dependence on an industrial infrastructure? The vast majority of farmers on the planet couldn't afford to buy the equipment and fertility that the green revolution crops demand. They lost their land and their communities lost their self-sufficiency. The swollen misery of Third World cities is a direct result. Draft horses and water buffalos require no steel mills, no fossil fuels, no bank loans. Even better: neither does a bison or an elk. But these options—sustainable, local, enmeshed in the processes of life—aren't even visible, let alone viable, to the political vegetarians, who want to save the world without ever knowing it.

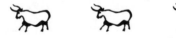

Why do we feed corn to cows? The corn will sicken them and, in turn, the humans who eat them.[38] So why do it? To answer that we need to understand farm policy in the United States. Farm policy is even more abstruse than the Haber-Bosch process, but we need to pursue it if we're going to make sense of why grass-eating ruminants are being stuffed with grain.

Between Fritz Haber and plant geneticists, the twentieth century saw corn yields increase from twenty-five bushels an acre to upward of one hundred and forty bushels an acre.[39] The United States alone produces ten billion bushels a year, and no matter how much liquid corn we swallow down in our Big Gulps, we'd never consume it all. Half of it is exported. Most of the remaining half goes into cows, pigs, and chickens. It costs a farmer $3 to grow a bushel, but it only fetches $2 "on what today passes for the open market."[40] The difference is paid by the federal government with enough extra to just keep the farmers in business.

This pattern was set during World War I. France became a battleground and English farmers had to be soldiers. It was up to the United States to feed our allies. "Plow to the fence for National Defense!" was the rallying cry of the federal government to US farmers. "For the first time, the federal government encouraged more production by setting minimum prices to be paid to farmers for basic food commodities," explains George Pyle.[41] After the war, those farmers, flush with cash, bought more land and more equipment. Tractors began to replace horses, freeing up more land for grain production, and the first hybrid seeds and chemical fertilizers appeared, raising production still further. Then Europe recovered and no longer needed food commodities from the United States. What all this meant was a huge surplus. What happened was an ever-growing pile of grain, which depressed prices, at the same time that the farmers, now heavily mortgaged, needed to earn cash. The Depression, "the existence of way too much stuff to buy and not enough money to buy it," hit the farm economy before the stock market crash in '29.[42] As farms went bust, the number of farmers tanked, "both in raw numbers—from 32.5 million to 30.5 million between 1916 and 1930—and as a percentage of the total population—from 32% to 25%."[43] With the

Great Depression in full swing, farm income plummeted 52 percent, and prices collapsed. Wheat fell from $1.30 to $0.38 a bushel, corn from $0.80 to $0.38.

A widget maker can reduce production if the market looks grim. This cuts her costs—raw materials, labor, energy—and the reduced supply of widgets will eventually drive the price back up. A farmer can't do this. First of all, the turnaround time for crops is too long to be responsive. Second, crops don't work like other inventory: you can't sell off the excess by dropping the price, as the prices are already lower than the cost of production, and they're set by international markets well beyond the farmer's control. In order for farmers to control prices, thousands of them would have to stop planting in concert to have any effect on the market.

Dropping the price doesn't spur an increase in consumption—people can only eat so much. Labor costs can't be reduced—most farms are already down to a one or two person operation: a pair of brothers, a husband and wife. Reducing the acreage planted would cut back a little on expenses for seed and fertilizer. But the overwhelming costs on a modern farm are fixed costs: the mortgage on the land and the equipment. So farmers are in a bind, which feels more like a noose. When prices are low, they need to produce even more to cover their fixed costs. But producing more only drives the prices lower. That's the situation that farmers find themselves in.

The point of the first federal farm price supports wasn't to make food available cheaply: it was to keep farmers in business. Because without farmers there is no food. And the free market doesn't work for basic foodstuffs. George Pyle, in his desperately important book *Raising Less Corn, More Hell*, explains:

> The woes of the farm economy were caused almost wholly
> by its collective habit of overproduction coupled with the
> individual farmer's inability to cut back on production and
> still have any income at all. The problem was not that we were
> running out of food ... [federal supports] existed to do the
> previously unthinkable. It paid farmers to produce less food.
> The idea was that if farm families could stay afloat, even for

a little while, on government payments, they would not be spurred to max out production just to keep from losing their farm to foreclosure.[44]

But the goal of limiting production to keep prices up was abandoned in the early 1970s. Michael Pollan explains that "instead of supporting farmers ... the government began supporting corn at the expense of farmers."[45]

The farm subsidies of the New Deal tried to keep prices up by allowing farmers to take loans with their crop as the loan guarantee. In surplus years, when prices were low and farmers would have gone bust, their grain was essentially sold to the government instead of being sold on the open market, where it would have driven prices lower still. Then when prices went up, the farmer could sell the grain. If the price swing took too long, the farmer could keep the loan and forfeit the crop. The government also sold the excess from its granary when drought or flood pushed prices up. This arrangement kept farmers on farms, and kept rural economies alive.

But in the 1970s, the New Deal programs were dismantled, replaced by a system of direct payments. The federal government pays subsidies to farmers if the price falls too low. Where before, corn was removed from the market when the price fell, now the market is continuously flooded.

The result has been an unending river of corn, drowning our arteries and our insulin receptors, our rural communities, and poor subsistence economies the world over. The corn comes at a huge environmental toll: there's a half gallon of oil in every bushel.[46] And it's essentially a massive transfer of money from the US taxpayer to the giant grain cartels, who are able to command the price of grain to be lower than the cost of production, with all of us making up the difference—five billion dollars in subsidies for corn alone, straight into the pockets of Cargill and Monsanto. [47]

We feed corn to cows because it's now cheap, though "we" isn't really a plural at all and certainly doesn't include the average citizen. Six firms control 75 percent of the grain handling facilities: they decide the price and farmers have to accept it. This condensation of control has moved up the commodity food chain: corn and soy are turned into cheap beef, pork, and chicken in an industrial process that can overlook entirely the fact that animals are living creatures. Some cultures consider feeding corn to animals a sacrilege; for corporate control of our food, it's a necessity.[48] Writes Michael Pollan, making a point that every free citizen should understand,

> [e]verything about corn meshes smoothly with the gears of this giant machine; grass doesn't. Grain is the closest thing in nature to an industrial commodity: storable, portable, fungible, ever the same today as it was yesterday and will be tomorrow. Since it can be accumulated and traded, grain is a form of wealth. It is a weapon, too ... The nation with the biggest surpluses of grain have always exerted power over the ones in short supply. Throughout history governments have encouraged their farmers to grow more than enough grain, to protect against famine, to free up labor for other purposes, to improve the trade balance, and generally to augment their own power ... The real beneficiary of this crop is not America's eaters but its military-industrial complex. In an industrial economy, the growing of grain supports the larger economy: the chemical and biotech industries, the oil industry, Detroit, pharmaceuticals (without which they couldn't keep animals healthy in CAFOs), agribusiness, and the balance of trade. Growing corn helps drive the very industrial complex that drives it. No wonder the government subsidizes it so lavishly.[49]

Having encouraged this orgy of cheap carbohydrates, the government then helped the grain cartels to use it by subsidizing CAFOs with tax relief, exempting them from environmental protection laws, and developing a meat grading system that elevated the fat "marbling" of grain-fed beef.

Now understand grass. Grass is not a commodity. It can't be easily stored, shipped, standardized, traded. It, like sunlight and rain, is the ultimate local, decentralized resource. And like sunlight and rain, it cannot lead to the condensation of power. Grass farmers need few if any fertilizers, pesticides, pharmaceuticals, fossil fuels. They aren't an industry—they are actual farmers, engaged in work that requires a skill set, not an instruction manual. Grass can't be turned into the hyper-processed cheap junk that fills our grocery stores. It can only be passed through a ruminant who will turn it into food, not a commodity, food as rooted as grass in a local ecology and a local economy.

And potentially a local politics. The populist movement was a movement of farmers: independent, ornery, proud, unbiddable. Now there aren't enough farmers left to fill a junior high school with progeny, let alone make common cause. The enemies are more structural than visible, though I'll point out that ADM and Monsanto have corporate headquarters and CEOs with addresses, and those corporations are responsible for the subsidies producing the oversupply, the collapsed prices, the extinction of small farmers the world over.

We feed corn to cows because corn is impossibly cheap, and feeding it to cows makes them grow fast, much faster than their native diet. A grain-fed steer reaches market weight in nine to twelve months instead of two years. CAFO chickens reach adulthood in six weeks rather than the five months they took in 1935, the heirloom speed for an heirloom farm.[50] A good milk cow in 1940 gave 4,500 pounds of milk a year. On grain, a dairy cow can produce in excess of 20,000.[51] Writes Michael Pollan, "So this is what commodity corn can do to a cow: industrialize the miracle of nature that is a ruminant, taking the sunlight- and prairie grass-powered organism and turning it into the last thing we need: another fossil fuel machine. This one, however, is able to suffer."[52]

The resulting product may be cheap, but there is a price to be paid, and we are all of us, animals, land, rivers, farmers, consumers, and citizens, paying it.

So you're an environmentalist; why are you supporting commodities instead of food, corporate profits over local, living economies, and power over justice?

Let's get specific. Cargill is the largest privately held corporation *on the planet.* Cargill and Continental each account for 25 percent of the grain trade: that's half between them.[53] Five companies control 75 percent of corn; four have a lock on 80 percent of global soybean processing.[54] "Farming is a pyramid," writes Richard Manning. "At the pinnacle ... stands ADM, the nation's largest buyer of grain."[55] They've flooded the world with cheap grain, and they've flooded the airwaves with their PR campaigns. You know the tagline: supermarket to the world. But do you understand what this tiny handful of companies is and what it's doing? They've driven prices down below production costs and kept them there. They've gotten the federal government— the US taxpayers—to make up the difference. They've destroyed small farms and local economies across the globe. And now, they own patents on the seeds themselves. Those seeds represent the knowledge, labor, and heritage of all of humanity, and their DNA is now *owned* by Monsanto and ConAgra and ADM. They're the oligarchs of food, the *pater familias* of life itself. "The ownership, genetic code, practices and profits of agriculture are being collected in fewer and fewer hands—hands that have no dirt under the fingernails," writes George Pyle.[56] And those hands owe nothing to anyone: not the starving children who have become a marketing cliche while they continue to starve; not the farmers, north, south, east, and west, who might have fed them but who are losing their farms. Nothing to anyone except, of course, the stockholders.

Read the labels on your soy milk and the groovy organic multigrain flakes you pour it on. Dean Foods owns White Wave/Silk. And the main shareholders of Dean Foods are: Citigroup, Coca-Cola, Exxon/Mobile, GE, Home Depot, Microsoft, Pfizer, Philip Morris, and Wal-Mart. Litelife, maker of the oh-so-righteous soy products served every year at my food co-op's annual member barbeque, is owned by ConAgra. Hain Food Group owns Bearitos, Bread Shop, Celestial Seasonings, Garden of Eatin', Health Valley, Imagine Foods (Rice Dream), Terra Chips, and Westbrae. And the prime investors in Hain Food Group are mutual funds and holding companies, with the principal stockholders being Citigroup, Entergy Nuclear (do I even need to continue?), Exxon/Mobil, weapons manufacturer Lockheed

Martin, Monsanto, Philip Morris, and to finish on a positive note, Wal-Mart. Cascadian Farms and Muir Glen are both owned by Small Planet Foods, which is owned by General Mills. And who "owns" General Mills? Alcoa Aluminium, Chevron, Disney, Dow Chemical, DuPont, Exxon/Mobil, General Electric, (vegetarians: take note) McDonald's, Monsanto, Nike, Pepsico, Philip Morris, Starbucks, Target Stores, and Texas Instruments (producer of weapons and George W. Bush). What else could I add to that list beside Voldemort? Meanwhile, CocaCola owns Fresh Samantha and Odwalla Juice, while Philip Morris owns Kraft Foods which owns Boca Burgers, and Nestle owns both Arrowhead Water and Poland Spring Water.[57]

Am I making my point?

So you're an environmentalist; why don't you know any of this?

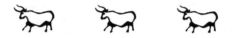

The trails of both cheap food commodities and political vegetarian ethics end in the same place: a starving child. She's the one we're supposed to be doing this for, our gluttony the cause of her suffering. Jim Motavalli continues, "As *Diet for a Small Planet* author Frances Moore Lappé writes, imagine sitting down to an 8 oz steak. 'Then imagine the room filled with 40-50 people with empty bowls in front of them. For the "feed cost" of your steak, each of their bowls could be filled with a full cup of cooked cereal grains.'"[58]

The "feed cost" of my steak could only feed the creatures that ate it, since it was mostly cellulose—grass and saplings—mixed in with mast, wild berries, insects. She's talking, as usual, about factory farming. Once again, set aside the considerations of climate and terrain, fertilizer and topsoil. Set aside as well that once the fossil fuel runs out, the grain will as well. Now understand: the surfeit of US grain and the starvation in poor countries *are not inverse, but proportional.*

Industrial farming—fossil fuels, genetics—created industrial yields. The size of those yields created factory farming, with surplus to spare. Those surpluses continue to grow because of the price-setting monopoly of three to six corporations, which fix prices below production, forcing farmers to produce ever more surplus to keep their land and their livelihoods. Those surpluses are then dumped in poor countries, wrecking their local subsistence economies, driving farmer-peasants off their land and into urban squalor. It may seem counterintuitive, but the last place to put cheap food is near chronically hungry people. Explains Lyle Vandyke, the former Canadian Minister of Agriculture:

> Consider a farmer in Ghana who used to be able to make a living growing rice. Several years ago, Ghana was able to feed [itself] and export their surplus. Now, it imports rice. From where? Developed countries. Why? Because it's cheaper. Even if it costs the rice producer in the developed world much more to produce the rice, he doesn't have to make a profit from his crop. The government pays him to grow it, so he can sell it more cheaply to Ghana than the farmer in Ghana can. And that farmer in Ghana? He can't feed his family anymore.[59]

Western countries support the giant food producers with subsidies totaling $360 billion. The effect "is overwhelmingly to reduce world prices."[60] According to Oxfam, "Exporters can offer US surpluses for sale at prices around half the cost of production; destroying local agriculture and creating a captive market in the process."[61]

In response, governments in poor countries try to erect trade barriers and tariffs. But those protective measures are being struck down in the name of free trade. For instance, the WTO ruled that the Philippine government must lower trade barriers to half their current levels over the next six years. This will effectively flood the Filipino market with cheap food commodities from the US and Europe. Oxfam predicts that the average farm income will drop by 30 percent as prices fall. Corn could end up selling for *less than half* its current price. There are 1.2 million Filipino maize farmers: as many as half a million "are under immediate threat."[62]

This cycle of corporate control, oversupply, and dumping leads to the destruction of local subsistence economies. It "undermines the livelihoods of 70 percent of the world's poorest people."[63] This is hardly a solution to world hunger.

And dismantling the current subsidy system—while not a bad idea—may not change much. According to the Agricultural Policy Analysis Center, "even the total elimination of US farm subsidies would result in only negligible increases in US prices for corn, wheat and soybeans ... The small price increase would then gradually decline to nothing over nine years, as the price rise encouraged new production, oversupply and a resulting price depression ... [D]umping would continue."[64]

Their answer? "Supply management is required." The exporting countries need to stop dumping, which means they need to stop producing surpluses. Practically, that means standing up to the corporations that literally own the food supply in the US. Politically, it requires understanding what has happened to turn food—our sustenance, our future—into a commodity. Chronic oversupply is the enemy of farmers in both rich and poor countries. *Grain from the US is causing starvation, not easing it.*

There is a severe schizophrenia on the Left. Anyone liberal to radical has some understanding that relationships of power cannot create justice. And justice is our North Star, our deepest wish. A colonial arrangement where the power center takes raw materials and cheap labor from the colony, destroying their local subsistence economies and their local land bases, is what we used to call "imperialism." Now we call it "globalization." No one calls it justice.

Except when it comes to food. Suddenly, we're aiming for exactly the above arrangement of power. But ask yourself: why should people in Cambodia be dependent on the US for their basic sustenance? It condemns them to participating in a market economy where they will have to dedicate their labor and local resources to produce raw materials, like timber and metal ore, or cheap consumer goods like sneakers or computer chips, for rich nations. With the pennies they get in return, they will then have to buy food from the same rich nations or their progeny, the grain cartels. This is a destructive, inhumane, and oppressive arrangement. I have to believe that the political vegetarians haven't thought it through.

So you're an environmentalist who wants to stop world hunger. Here's what you should do.

Try everything in your power to stop the grain cartels, including revoking their corporate charters. Then understand how federal farm policies are driving local economies into ruin and farmers into suicide the world over. I know it's Byzantine and boring, but get involved in local, state, and national campaigns to change those policies. There are also human rights, feminist, and pro-democracy movements in poor countries who could use our money and our help. Ultimately, the overlapping subsets of globalization, capitalism, industrialization, and patriarchy have got to be confronted and dismantled. Nothing less will create a just and sustainable world.

Refraining from factory farm animal products is a righteous act, for animals and the earth, but it will not feed a single hungry person. The hungry don't have the money to buy North American grain; getting the money means further dependence on the masters of globalization; and cheap commodities from afar only further destroy local food production, the only real food security that can exist. This is why there are *no* international aid agencies that suggest vegetarianism as a solution to world hunger: it isn't one. I understand how the desperate longing for a just and fed world can lead us to cling to simple answers, especially answers that are easy to institute in our personal lives. But buying a soy burger is an emotional quick fix that does not address the tenacious and terrible roots of power and inequality. Check the label: you're probably giving money to the very corporations that are creating the problem.

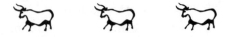

The pursuit of a just, sustainable, and local economy will eventually lead us to the grim conclusion that there are simply too many of us. The world population is supposed to reach 8.9 billion by 2050.[65] Meanwhile the oceans will be fished empty by 2050, the aquifers and water tables will be well out of reach, and the last trace of topsoil rendered dust. We are already living on fossil fuel and this—right now—is the historical moment when oil will peak. It will never be this cheap or accessible again. What then?

We are a species on overshoot, and we have been for ten thousand years. Each level of technology that we've achieved has only accelerated the problem, both by increasing our population and by increasing our consumption. A citizen of the United States, for instance, consumes fifty-seven times more than a citizen of India. "The average American produces the same greenhouse-gas emissions as four and a half Mexicans, or 18 Indians, or 99 Bangladeshis," writes Elizabeth Colbert.[66] No rational person could honestly believe that our finite planet can provide for this way of life indefinitely, even when so few of us have it, and especially when there are so many more who want it.

There are pitfalls to talking about overpopulation, the most serious being racism. People with a racist agenda have used the idea of overpopulation to fuel their heinous goals, and we need to face that squarely. We also need to face that our planet cannot support our existing numbers even at subsistence levels. We are drawing down stored resources—the natural capital of the earth—and when the oil, soil, fish, and water are gone, we will starve.

The concept of carrying capacity is crucial to any discussion of population. William Catton, in his critically important book *Overshoot*, writes:

> It has now become essential to recognize that all creatures, human or otherwise, impose a load upon their environment's ability to supply what they need and to absorb and transform what they excrete or discard. An environment's carrying capacity for a given kind of creature (living a given way of life) is the *maximum persistently feasible load*—just short of the load that would damage that environment's ability to support life of that kind. Carrying capacity can be expressed quantitatively as the number of us, living in a given manner, which a given environment can support *indefinitely*.[67]

The first method humans used to increase our population was displacement: we took over a spot in the food chain occupied by someone else. There's nothing immoral, destructive, or unique in this activity. It's simply what every species does, how evolution works. A new life form evolves that can use a niche better than anyone else. In the process, other species are supplanted and die out. Eventually the new species will become the old, to be replaced in its turn as climates change, food supplies shift, and competitors evolve. This is the long trajectory of life, from self-organizing proteins to redwoods and red wings.

Tree-dwelling primates developed opposable thumbs for grasping branches. They dropped to the ground and kept their thumbs, and they had brains just big enough to use the prototype tool: a rock. Some researchers believe we became human by using brains, our own and those of our scavenged or hunted food. Other animals can't get into the skull case of prey. The simple act of lifting and smashing down a rock opened the skull and the nutrient-dense brains within. We don't eat brains in the US; only the culturally unassimilated still eat organ meats of any kind. But organ meats hold the most nutrition, and brains are especially rich in fatty acids. "[T]he ability to use the hands allowed early human and prehuman ancestors to obtain essential fats found in large concentrations in the brains of other animals, an area pretty much off-limits to other carnivores because of the thickness of the bony skull."[68] Note that the human brain is over 60 percent fat. We used our brains to create more of the same, which in turn has let us displace species all over the world. Our ability to make fire, shelter, clothing, enabled us to leave the tropics, our original home, and a great number of our microfaunal predators.

In the process we displaced other species. "Human tribes," explains Stewart Udall, "took over for human use portions of the life-supporting potential of the biosphere that would otherwise have sustained other forms of life."[69]

Agriculture is another level entirely. Instead of occupying a niche inside an ecosystem, humans occupied entire ecosystems, turning biotic communities into monocrops, as we have seen. Explains Catton, each enlargement of carrying capacity ... consisted essentially of *diverting* some fraction of the earth's life-supporting capacity from supporting other kinds of life to supporting our kind. Our pre-*sapiens* ancestors, with their simple stone tools and fire, took over for human use organic materials that would otherwise have been consumed by insects, carnivores, or bacteria. From about 10,000 years ago, our earliest horticulturalist ancestors began taking over *land* upon which to grow crops for human consumption. That land would otherwise have supported trees, shrubs, or wild grasses, and all the animals dependent thereon—but fewer humans. As the expanding generations replaced each other, *Homo sapiens* took over more and more of the surface of this planet, essentially at the expense of its other inhabitants.[70]

Instead of sustaining ourselves inside a complex web of relationships, we destroyed those relationships, taking the land and the sunlight for ourselves.

There are other species who change their ecosystems dramatically. Beavers, for instance, will eat their way through acres of riparian forest and dam entire rivers. The difference is that beavers, with their engineering skills, create wetlands, the most diverse habitat on the planet, while humans have created deserts and dead zones with our technologies.

Actually, any species that outstrips its natural checks will overshoot its environment. In this way we are no different than the bacteria in a wine barrel. With nothing to stop them, the bacteria reproduce at an exponential rate until they use up their entire food store. Then they die, poisoned by their own waste products. Catton points out that "[t]he same kind of thing happens in a pond when its plant and animal inhabitants fill it with organic debris and turn it into a meadow, in which aquatic creatures can no longer live."[71] This is a natural process called *succession*. "Organisms using their habitat unavoidably reduce its capacity to support their kind by what they necessarily do to it in the process of living. In making their habitat less suitable for themselves, organisms sometimes make it more suitable for other species—their successors."[72]

Beavers can move on, and over the course of centuries the cycle of wetlands turning to meadows and forests and then back to beaver will repeat itself. Wine vat microorganisms, on the other hand, have nowhere else to go. Likewise, the famous deer on St. Matthew Island: without predators, an original population of twenty-nine deer peaked at six thousand, then crashed to forty-two, leaving a permanently degraded habitat.[73] Like the deer, humans found and then filled new territory—every continent except Antarctica—that was mostly free from the small, hungry things that set up residence in human tissue in the tropics. What Catton calls the "takeover" method of human expansion has reached an end: there are no new continents left to take.

What humans have turned to is the "drawdown" method, using nonrenewable resources instead of new territory to increase our numbers.

> About 1800 A. D., a new phase in the ecological history of humanity began. Carrying capacity was tremendously (but temporarily) augmented by a quite different method; takeover gave way to drawdown. A conspicuous and unprecedentedly large acceleration of human population increase got under way as *Homo sapiens* began to supersede agrarian living with industrial living.[74]

Coal-fueled machinery allowed irrigation, enhanced agricultural production, and transported foodstuffs. Coal gave way to oil and gas, and the horse's day was done.[75] The one-quarter to one-third of agricultural land that had been dedicated to draft animals could now grow humans. And finally the Haber-Bosch process exploded onto the world.

The massive population shift from food-producers in rural areas to food-consuming, industrial-producers in urban areas has resulted in a profound level of ignorance of where our food comes from, what its necessary inputs are, and what toll it's taking on the landbase. This ignorance means that each culture, each bioregion, each individual has no basis to make a reasoned judgment of her impact on planetary health even while our planet is dying.

Take a country like Japan. According to Catton, if the Japanese weren't relying on fisheries around the world and trade with agriculture-exporting nations, two-thirds of the country would be starving.[76] Likewise, in Great Britain, over half of the country's food comes from outside its borders, with 6.5 percent from the sea and 48 percent from other countries.[77] There are clearly more people in those countries than the land can support. What they are living on is "ghost acreage." This is a concept developed by Georg Borstrom in his book *The Hungry Planet*. A country's farms, pastures, and forests are their "visible acres." The "ghost acres" are the food sources beyond its borders. Once the carrying capacity of the country is reached, more people can only be fed by using imports from ghost acres. Ghost acreage can be further divided into "fish acreage"—food from the oceans—and "trade acreage"—food from countries that export agricultural products. This is the situation of most countries: they're dependent on a very few grain-exporting nations.

Because there's no mass starvation in Japan or Britain and the stores are filled with staples, no one realizes that they've collectively overshot their locality, their bioregion, their country. No one needs to. Since the food doesn't grow where we live—what can grow in cement and between parked cars?—we don't see the cost: the dead zones and desperate terns. There's no after-image of a once-living prairie burned on our retinas as we gaze down on the flyover states. Even our mythic matrix contains no point of reference to what we've devoured: whole continents that other creatures once knew as home, wiped to the clean bone of monocultures. And because we don't grow the food ourselves, we have no idea that our current numbers are only possible through cheap fossil fuel.

Our dependence on oil, gas, and coal produces what Catton names a "phantom carrying capacity." It's not a true carrying capacity—the environment cannot support these numbers indefinitely, only until the fossil fuels run out. To fish and trade acreage, Catton adds the concept of "fossil acreage," which he defines as "the number of additional acres of farmland that would have been needed to grow organic fuels with equivalent energy content."[78] The concept of fossil acreage is harder for most people to grasp than fish or trade acres, which become self-evident to anyone who can do basic arithmetic. But the idea of "fossil acres" requires a knowledge base—essentially of the nature of nature, versus the nature of annual monocrops—that industrial urbanites lack.

This is true even for honorable, earnest people who want justice and sustainability. Jim Merkel in his book *Radical Simplicity* ends up urging the typical vegan diet. The math is simple: "There are 28.2 billion acres of bioproductive land—the total surface area minus the deep oceans, deserts, icecaps and built-up land."[79] Divided by six billion people equals 4.7 acres for each of us. Of course that excludes every other living thing. To protect biodiversity and species viability, between 25-75 percent of total land in most areas would have to be put in reserves with buffer zones.[80] Through various calculations the reader can choose how big of an "Ecological Footprint" (EF) they want to take for their food. Merkel then walks us through a 0.4 acre food EF, a 1.2 acre EF, and a 1.6 acre food EF.

Set aside that all his numbers for animal products are, of course, factory farmed and grain fed, which, I agree, is wasteful, destructive, and cruel. *There is no way that acreage that small can feed a human being.* The only reason that 5 billion people have any food is that we've displaced vast numbers of species and we're eating fossil fuel. The nitrogen for this food is being manufactured from gas and oil, and we are on a crash course with reality. Jim Merkel and many good people like him are failing to face the full extent of the problem, not for lack of courage, but for lack of information.

For instance, he writes, "in the case of a .4 acre food EF, this sample person grows 60 lbs. of their monthly veggies, potatoes, and fruit on 256 square yards of fair soil. They had plenty of food, about 2.6 lbs. a day, but a slim condiment bar."[81]

Plenty of food maybe, but what they also had was plenty of malnutrition. "With ... some grains, beans and eggs, this person's energy and dietary needs could be met," he adds.

This diet is never going to provide enough protein, fat, fat soluble vitamins, or minerals for long term maintenance and repair of the human body. Bulk calories, yes, but this is a poverty diet, as half-starved people the world over can attest to with their small and arthritic skeletons, their exhaustion, their pellagra, and their orange hair. And so can their blind and retarded children.

But never mind that for now. The real question is, what is going to fertilize that .4 acre garden? You don't get something from nothing. Every pound of happy veggies he harvests means minerals and nitrogen mined from the soil. Unless he's using permanent mulch (which comes from where?) and some animal bones, blood, manure (also unaccounted for in his numbers), the soil, organism by organism, will eventually die, collapsing into dust. And *grains?* Merkel lives in Vermont.

Meanwhile, down the road is a small family dairy farm, hanging on by its Carhartt fingernails. They may have gotten sucked into the factory farm model as milk prices dropped below production costs. But Merkel could easily find one nearby that stuck to its guns—heirloom cows on grass. He could forget the starvation rations and the annual monocrops, and instead eat what grows sustainably where he lives: animals integrated into a perennial polyculture. He could actually be fed. A thousand years from now, Merkel's descendants will have long since abandoned his devastated garden plot. Meanwhile the dairy farmer's line—including the cows—will have produced food while growing a few more inches of topsoil, verdant with the partnerships between animals and plants, humans and cows, soil and all of us.

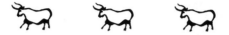

We're asking the wrong question. It's for the right reasons: we want a just world where every last child is fed. But our species overshot a long time ago and *it can't be done.* In the end, phantom carrying capacity can produce only ghosts, and they will be hungry ones. We're using up fossil acres, harvesting sunlight that's been stored away for thousands of years. Once it's gone, there won't be any more. "Facts are not repealed by refusal to face them," writes Catton.[82] We—human race we—are going to have to face the facts if we have any hope of easing our way toward true sustainability while valuing human rights and preserving civic order. The alternative is a grim and ugly scenario of mass starvation, plagues, racial and tribal strife, misogyny, fundamentalism, and accelerating ecosystem collapse. *Mad Max* meets *The Handmaid's Tale* in the *Soylent Green* Café?

I don't believe in the rapture. This planet is my home. I want a culture that cherishes the earth with reverence and awe and that by necessity respects the limits we must impose on ourselves. My hope—and it's an increasingly desperate one as the ice sheets melt—is that we can willingly embrace those limits once we understand that the planet is finite and the fossil fuel is running out. Otherwise the crash is going to be ugly.

It is not my project to try to feed every human being that we can produce while we chew the planet to the bone. I'm not asking, *How many people can be fed?* but a very different question: How *can* people be fed? Not, *What feeds the most people?* but *What feeds people sustainably?* We need a full accounting. The absolute bottom line is: what methods of food production build topsoil while using only ambient sun and rain? *Because nothing else is sustainable.* To quote George Draffan, "I'll repeat the obvious: sustainable systems are the only ones that are sustainable."[83] Using those methods, and only those methods, how many humans can the planet support? Because the day we produce one more of us is the day we need to be ashamed of ourselves as a species.

William Catton and other peak oil writers think that our numbers overshot in 1800 CE. That year stands in as the beginning of the fossil fuel age. We began to produce increasing amounts of food by using reserves of energy that were nonreplicating, nonrenewable. I agree that the year 1800 marks a change in human culture and consumption that has been profoundly destructive. But I would push the beginning of the drawdown age back about ten thousand years, to the beginning of agriculture. What I am proposing is the concept of *fossil soil*. Soil is an ancient biological reserve that we have been destroying ever since we became dependent on annual grains. Explains Steven Stoll:

> Lost soil is unrecoverable, and the pace of its formation is so
> slow that the end product must be considered nonrenewable.
> One survey of a southern district in the 1930s found earth-
> works abandoned on land not cultivated since 1887. Under
> the pine crowns, on high ground, the researchers found fifty
> years of accumulated topsoil one-sixteenth of an inch deep. At
> that rate of creation the pines would see their first inch in eight
> hundred years, their first foot in ninety-six hundred years—the
> age of agriculture itself. In human time it can be lost forever....
> Subsoils are the bones of the earth. They have no living organ-
> isms and no rotting plant food, and they hold little water. All
> these are lost with topsoils, and people follow.[84]

That destruction meant that human numbers could increase—
but only by decimating habitat, ecosystems, and ultimately the soil.
A population that relies on a drawdown of *the basis of life itself* cannot
be sustained. This should be self-evident, but it's been ten thousand
years and we're clearly not catching on. Jim Merkel hasn't; neither has
the permaculture crew in upstate New York with their diet of wheat
and soy. And those are people who are trying, who want a just and
living world, and who are willing to make enormous personal sacrifices toward that end.

For instance, Merkel writes that "[p]asture is the land where
animals graze, providing meat, hides, wool and milk.... [It] is less
productive than cropland."[85] Remember that two-thirds of the earth's
land is unsuited for annual grain crops, including his home state of
Vermont, with its cold climate, thin, acid soil, and steep terrain. This
is one of the main reasons why his Ecological Footprint (EF) is of
limited value when it comes to food: what grows where he lives—and
grows sustainably—is given a *higher* (worse) EF than food that is both
from far away and that is ultimately destructive. "Less productive"
for whom? Bison, salmon, frogs? What is productive about destroying Mesopotamia, Sindh, the Great Plains forever? It may temporarily
produce more calories for humans, but only by exterminating plants
and animals, applying nitrogen made from natural gas, and drawing
down the fossil soil.

Merkel references some truly sustainable cultures. He describes the Chumash, whose traditional territory is around San Luis Obispo, California. Their traditional foods included acorns, pine nuts, deer, bear, rabbit, birds, fresh and saltwater fish, clams, fruits, mushrooms, and tubers. When the Spanish arrived, there were 25,000 people in eighty-five villages. There were also other apex predators—grizzlies, mountain lions—a clear indication that they were not overshooting their land base. "The Chumash had a sustainable lifestyle," he writes.[86] He sees that their matrilineal structure and communal ethic of non-accumulation are key components of their sustainable lifeway. He doesn't see that the food he is promoting is the *exact opposite* of theirs. They ate the plants and animals that lived within their local forests, rivers, and seacoasts—within nature's basic pattern of animals integrated into perennial polycultures. Yet he wants us to eat annual monocrops with no animal inputs, food that requires biotic cleansing and is only made possible by drawing down unnoticed and unnamed reserves of fossil soil and fossil fuel. Whether we see them now or not, we will certainly notice them when they're gone.

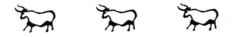

How many people can the planet support? If you use 1800 CE as your benchmark, there were roughly 1 billion people at the start of the fossil fuel age. If you use 8000 BCE—the beginning of agriculture—there were about 8 million of us at the start of the fossil soil age. The population of the Americas hadn't reached carrying capacity at that point. We need to add that in. This may be honestly impossible as estimates on American numbers at European contact vary widely and bitterly. The high counters say sixty million; the low say two million. Some middle ground experts say eighteen million. We will probably never know. One thing we do know is that once agriculture was established in the Americas, it followed the same pattern of population overshoot and environmental degradation among the Aztec, the Mayans, the Anasazi, the mound-building Cahokia, the cities that DeSoto found along the Gulf Coast from present day Florida to

Louisiana. There was deforestation in both the north and south east along the coast and along the major rivers, and overpopulation pressures, created ultimately by sedentary, civilized corn cultures. Whatever the number was by 1492, in some places it was already too high.

Merkel, who wants to make room for the animals and the wild, for the rest of our siblings, suggests 600 million as a sustainable number. My guess is his number is way too high; the fossil fuel and fossil soil aren't visible to him, or to the political vegetarians he's drawing his calculations from. My number would be much lower. But does it matter in the end what number I come up with? There needs to be fewer of us. Dramatically fewer of us. And in wealthy countries, we need to consume dramatically less. A truly local economy could make that necessity both plain and possible: not only would it be obvious that logging, mining, agriculture, and other extractive activities were necessary for our McMansions and our computer chips, but when those "resources" ran out, so would the life that is built upon them. But money buys us distance, buffering us from the murder of the world in a sweet dream of abundance.

Brian Donahue explores this in his book *Reclaiming the Commons: Community Farms and Forests in a New England Town.* The town of Weston has a community-owned forest, and the question of human use has proved difficult. He writes, "If we face a future in which fossil fuel use must be cut dramatically to avoid bringing the ecological disasters of poisoned air and disrupted climate down on forests ... it seems inescapable that we must turn to the local biological resources immediately surrounding us to meet a larger proportion of our needs."[87] He continues more pointedly,

> we must have a functional connection with nature to live. Most environmentalists ... are affluent people whose consumption of forest products is large. How can this be reconciled with the idea that we should refrain from managing our own forests productively? Why should we enjoy this luxury, unless we baldly state the truth that we would rather such unseemly extraction take place somewhere else, out of sight?[88]

Human life, like all life, requires resources. But the link between cause and effect, between consumption and degradation, has been broken in our cultural consciousness. If we had to draw our sustenance from our local foodshed, instead of across continents and sold to the highest bidder, we would notice when our activities and our numbers were degrading our land base. Our empty stomachs, for instance, would be happy to tell us.

This is why hunter-gatherers are much better at keeping their populations in check. Overexploiting a food source leads to starvation in a very quick season or two. Agriculture, on the other hand, increases human numbers through the very act of destroying the landbase. Writes Toby Hemenway,

> when a forest is cleared for crops the loss of biodiversity translates into more food for people. Soil begins to deplete immediately but that won't be noticed for many years. When the soil is finally ruined, which is the fate of nearly all agricultural soils, it will stunt ecological recovery for decades. But while the soil is steadily eroding, crops will support a growing village.... Forager cultures have a built-in check since the plants and animals they depend on cannot be over-harvested without immediate harm, but ... [t]here are no structural constraints on agriculture's ecologically damaging tendencies."[89]

This is not to romanticize life in a hunter-gatherer culture. Infanticide was the fallback plan for excess numbers. Most cultures had herbal contraceptives and abortifacients, but those aren't terribly effective. Breast-feeding is often toted as hunter-gatherer birth control, but it's only about 80 percent reliable. Lactation will stop a woman's menses, but she may still ovulate—which means she can still conceive. For comparison, the rhythm method is also 80 percent effective, and, as many Catholic women can attest, 80 percent can mean a baby a year.

Many cultures embrace taboos on sexual intercourse for parents of children under five, or have a special role for celibate and homosexual people. But an Inuit woman whose husband died was expected to kill any children under the age of three: in a severe climate, the ratio between adults and dependents is that delicate.[90] I can't believe it was any easier for a woman in that world to kill her child than it would be for us. Survival sometimes requires brutal actions.

Some cultures had a different view of sexual intercourse altogether. Semen is believed to contain a life force that strengthens a man if kept and weakens him if spent. Explains Carolyn Niethammer, "Although there was little of the prudishness and prurience often found in conjunction with sex in [Euro-]American or Western European society, there was a deep-seated feeling in many [North American] tribes that the sex act diminished certain male powers."[91] In some militaristically patriarchal cultures, like the Melanesian Islands, semen is passed from older men to younger in religious rituals, while sexual intercourse with women is considered a duty for procreation, to be avoided as much as possible.[92]

Like almost everything that humans do, sex is a social institution. Who does it, why they do it, how they do it: the answers are shaped by the culture we live in. Right now, patriarchy is the ruling religion of the planet. The brute facts are that most women in the world have no control over the uses to which men put their bodies, sexually or reproductively. The chairman of the World Health Organization's AIDS meeting declared that male-dominated societies are a health threat across the planet.[93] When masculinity is built around a violation imperative, when male identity claims a right to access and dominate whatever it wants—be that women's bodies, wilderness, or the genetic code—the results will be rape, AIDS and unwanted pregnancies, environmental devastation, and a science built on the breaking of boundaries.[94] Women the world over need access to contraception and abortion, but they also need liberty. That liberty will only be won when masculinity—its religion, its economics, its psychology, its sex—is resisted and defeated.

Have I fallen off the map of the known world? Should I care when the world is dying?

So you're an environmentalist; become a cartographer of freedom.

I want to be clear. I'm not arguing that all non-industrial or even non-agricultural cultures are intrinsically egalitarian. They aren't. Social hierarchies based on sex, race (I'm counting xenophobia as proto-racism), age, or status exist in many hunter-gatherer cultures. Plenty of cultures with sustainable lifeways practiced torture, rape, war, even genocide. These are separate social phenomena from material sustainability. Sometimes they overlap; in other cultures they don't.[95]

No matter how sustainable the material culture, when men have the power, women and girls are their property, to be bought and sold, traded, loaned, and given away.[96] Women who commit or are even suspected of adultery in such cultures may be subject to rape, public stripping and whipping, disfigurement, torture, and murder.[97]

And then there's female hunger. Anthropologist Magdalena Hurtado lived with the Ache, hunter-gatherers in the tropical rainforest of Paraguay. She assumed that hunter-gatherers were egalitarian and that food was shared by all. She learned very quickly how wrong that assumption was. Among the Ache, married women are completely dependent on their husbands for meat: it was up to each individual man whether or how much to share. Not only that, but the food that the women collected *also* belonged to their husbands. The women could only eat after the men had taken what they wanted. As well as the chronic hunger, Hurtado got to experience firsthand the food obsession and food-hoarding behaviors of the Ache women. She quips, "While ceasing to eat, I worked to convince myself of the merits of cultural relativism."[98]

Susan Allport comments, "Men in many societies restrict the amount of resources that their wives can use—even food resources. Food taboos are common throughout the world, in both hunter-gatherer and agricultural societies, and the most common taboos involve what and when women are allowed to eat."[99] Among the Chipewyans, women only ate after the men took what they wanted, which meant they often got nothing.[100] In regions of Africa and southern Asia, women's work includes caring for chickens, yet men forbid them to eat either chickens or eggs. In parts of Indonesia, all meat belongs to men. Allport continues, "'Being women, eat crumbs' is a saying among the Chuckee of the northern extreme of Siberia, where women eat only after their husbands have eaten and have taken the choicest parts of the food. The sharing practices of the Australian Aborigines—where the order of preference in food distribution is old men, hunting men, children, dogs, and women—blatantly prevent women from eating animal fat most of their lives."[101]

Old men, hunting men, children, dogs, and women: if that's not a hierarchy, what is? Besides the suffering of chronic hunger, such food restrictions are responsible for female malnutrition and increased mortality, especially among pregnant and lactating women.

Meanwhile, in modern North America, 40 percent of nine-year-old girls have dieted and 9 percent of them have vomited to lose weight. 81 percent of ten-year-olds have dieted and the number one wish of girls 11-17 years old is to lose weight.[102] Anorexia "has the highest mortality rate of any mental illness—up to 20%."[103]

For most women in our industrial, media-saturated culture, every meal has been turned into a tightrope strung between self-loathing and chronic hunger: at any given moment, 70 percent of women are on a diet and "40% are continually gaining and losing weight."[104] Eating disorders are now the third most common chronic illness in adolescent girls.[105] In fact, "the annual death rate associated with anorexia is more than *12 times higher* than the annual death rate due to *all* other causes combined for females between 15 and 24 years old."[106]

Statements about the egalitarian nature of indigenous hunter-gatherer or non-industrial societies need to be contextualized, and everybody human has to count.[107] Many settled coastal peoples, for instance, develop "Big Man" societies. One man is the identified leader and his status is increased by lavish acts of generosity, and even waste. Such displays may include the public killing of slaves as a conspicuous display of wealth. Just because they honored the fish and forests, doesn't mean that sustainable cultures honored human rights. A given people's approach to their sustenance and their landbase says nothing about whether men brutalize women, or whether the stranger is tortured—torture that could include slow evisceration or being burned alive for hours—or fed.

A culture's material sustainability also does not answer to how they treated animals. Some hunter-gatherers kept captured birds in tiny cages for eggs and meat. Then there's fire, the tool that catapulted humans from dwellers in the land to shapers of the land. Fire for hunting, for ecosystem management, and for communication may be a sustainable tool, but it can be unfathomably cruel. One observer saw "whole herds of Buffaloes with their hair singed—some were blind; and half roasted carcasses strewed our way." Another described "blind buffalo ... seen every moment wandering off ... The poor beasts have all their hair singed off; even skin in many places is shriveled up and terribly burned, and their eyes are swollen and closed fast. It was really pitiful to see them staggering about, sometimes running afoul of a large stone, at other times tumbling down hill and falling into creeks not yet frozen over." Other observers speak of "deer, elk, buffaloes, and wolves dead from fires, of herds of up to one thousand animals killed, and of thousands of beavers immolated."[108] No sentient being should have to endure this, and a human culture worth the name should not countenance it. These issues of universal human rights, of animal rights, of how compassion and respect intersect (or not) with cultural diversity, are of profound importance. But they tell us nothing about a culture's impact on its land base.

People who characterize hunter-gatherer cultures as "egalitarian" are getting at something, however much is missing from that description. Because agricultural societies, and only agricultural societies, develop civilizations, centralized hierarchies of control. This process is universal. It happened everywhere agriculture took root, and the reason is surplus. Toby Hemenway explains:

> The damage done by agriculture is social and political as well.
> A surplus, rare and ephemeral for foragers, is a principal goal

of agriculture. A surplus must be stored, which requires technology and materials to build storage, people to guard it, and a hierarchical organization to centralize the storage and decide how it will be distributed. It also offers a target for local power struggles and theft by neighboring groups, increasing the scale of wars. With agriculture, power thus begins its concentration into fewer and fewer hands. He who controls the surplus controls the group. Personal freedom erodes naturally under agriculture. [109]

Or, as Richard Manning puts it, "Agriculture was not so much about food as it was about the accumulation of wealth. It benefited some humans, and those people have been in charge ever since."[110]

These centralized hierarchies put the bulk of the population at the bottom of the social pyramid. Remember, 80 percent of the population was in slavery or serfdom in the year 1800. Why? Because agriculture requires backbreaking labor; agriculturalists need surplus because they're sedentary (hunter-gatherers simply move on when they're out of food); enslaving that many people requires an army to keep them enslaved; the surplus produced needs an army to store and protect it; and the destruction of land necessitates imperialist expansion, which needs an army and the surplus to feed it—i.e., more agriculture. If this all seems circular, it is. It's a feedback loop that's been spinning ever faster for ten thousand years, sucking in people, cultures, and ecosystems, while spitting out starvation and destruction.

Forget all the definitions of civilization involving "good breeding; politeness; consideration." The most basic root of civilization—both the word and the process—is the city. A city means people gathered in numbers that the landbase could never support. It requires agriculture, which is the destruction of biotic communities. Derrick Jensen distinguishes civilization from camps and villages by defining cities "as people living more or less permanently in one place in densities high enough to require the routine importation of food and other necessities."[111] The point of his book *Endgame* is that civilization will never be sustainable, and he's right: it won't be. For food to be imported to cities necessitates agriculture and its attendant surplus.

As we have seen, agriculture is the drawdown of fossil soil and the monocropping of continents. But agriculture is also the devastation of human culture. The myth of civilization is that it creates security, when what it creates is centralized social hierarchy and systematic hunger. Richard Manning points out that by making wealth possible, agriculture also invented poverty.[112] "Famine is a creation of farming," he writes, then details the millions of people who have starved over the last six thousand years. These details swell with horror. In 200 BCE, half of China's population died of hunger. The emperor legalized the eating and selling of children as meat.[113] To the argument that world hunger is a political problem of distribution, Manning answers that "poverty is agriculture's chief product."[114]

The myth is that civilization has been a net plus for human rights and human happiness. Since history belongs to the victors, that is what the civilized would say—but *they* are the ones who owned the slaves, the rest of us. Those slaves have been what made the rulers' leisure and luxury, philosophy and art, possible. Athens, the mighty birthplace of capital-D Democracy, was 90 percent slaves. Wrote South Carolina Senator William Harper in 1837, "[T]he institution of Slavery is a principal cause of civilization. Perhaps nothing can be more evident than that it is the sole cause.... Without it, there can be no accumulation of property, no providence for the future, no taste for comforts or elegancies, which are the characteristics and essentials of civilization.... Servitude is the condition of civilization."

We are living in that brief historical moment when cheap fossil fuel has made unimaginable consumption possible. Of all the goods ever produced, half of them have been made and consumed since 1950. But if the energy provided by fossil fuel to support the average inhabitant of the US had to be produced by human power, we would each have 120 slaves.[115] To grind the grain of the civilized, female slaves spent their lives bent over on hands and knees, leaving their arthritic and deformed legs and spines to speak to us in silent outrage. Are you listening? Agricultural foods—the grains, beans, and vegetables we are all urged to eat in the service of world community—are the foods of displacement and destruction, not justice or peace. They have been the foods of slavery, and when this short moment of oil engorgement fades into memory and then into myth, we will be left with sweat. The only choice will be whether that sweat is our own or our slaves'. Grain requires sweat. The planet wants to be a living community, not a monocrop. Just as war needs soldiers, the civilized need slaves. It is no good insisting we will somehow do it better in the post-carbon future. Agricultural food is soaked clean through in oil and blood. Take the fossil fuel out of the equation and tell me where there is room left for human rights.

From the beginning, "farming spread by genocide."[116] When the LBK agriculturalists (linearbandkeramik, after their decorative pottery) migrated from their origins in southern Turkey to Europe, the hunter-gatherer Cro-Magnons were already living there. The archaeological record shows no trade between these people, no transfer of goods, with one exception: spear points. Writes Richard Manning, "And there is no reason to believe that they were exchanged in a nonviolent manner."[117] Civilization follows the same pattern everywhere. The only question is who will be displaced, who immiserated? This is the question that political vegetarians need to face and then answer.

Agriculture—its foods, its civilizations—is the end of the world. There is no peace in the warfare that agriculture demands, no justice in the slavery it requires, no life in the bare, salted rock it leaves behind. And there is nowhere else to go. These are our choices, as bare as that dead rock: accept our place as animals, a place both humble and wild, or impose ourselves and our food across our living home of land and sea and sky until the planet dies.

CHAPTER 4
Nutritional Vegetarians

Start with Africa seven million years ago, because that's where human life began. The climate, the creation of our ancestors—our beloved kin of bacteria, fungi, and plants—eased from wet to dry. The trees gave way to grasses and a tide of savannas rippled across the world. Cradled in the grasses were large herbivores. Twenty-five million years ago, in the exuberance of evolution, a few plants tried growing from their bases instead of their tips. Grazing would not kill these plants; quite the opposite. It would encourage them by stimulating root growth. All plants want nitrogen and predigested nutrients, and ruminants could provide those to the grasses as they grazed. This is why, unlike other plants, grasses contain no toxins or chemical repellents, no mechanical deterrents like thorns or spines to discourage animals. Grasses want to be grazed. It was grass that created cows; human "domestication" was, in comparison, just the tiniest tug on the bovine genome, and cows tugged back with the lactose tolerance gene.

Our direct line lived in trees, until the trees began to disappear. We had two evolutionary edges to see us through: our opposable thumbs and our omnivorous digestion. We had the capacity to manipulate tools and we had bodies equipped with both the instincts and the digestion to handle a range of foods. Some animals are monofeeders: koalas eat only eucalyptus, and fig wasps dine only on figs. Monofeeding is a gamble; if your food source fails, you go down with it. But a brain, which is a huge energy sink, can be small for a monofeeder, which spares energy for every other function.

Chocolate notwithstanding, humans are not monofeeders. Back before we were human, when we were tree dwellers, we ate mainly fruit, leaves, and insects. But from the moment we stood upright, we've been eating large ruminants. Four million years ago, Australopithecines, our species' forerunners, ate meat.

Australopithecines were once believed to be fruitivores: the dividing line between the Homo genus and Australopithecines was thought to be the taste for meat. But the teeth of four three-million-year-old skeletons in a South African cave told a different story. Anthropologists Matt Sponheimer and Julia Lee-Thorp found Carbon-13 in the tooth enamel of those skeletons. Carbon-13 is a stable isotope present in two places: grasses and the bodies of animals that eat grass. Those teeth showed none of the scratch marks of grass consumption.[1]

Australopithecine was eating grass-feeding animals, the large ruminants swaddled in savanna.

Stone tools have laid beside the bones of long-extinct animals, buried in a silence of time, for 2.6 million years. Together, tools and bones have waited to tell their story, the story of us. Some of the bones show teeth marks overlaid by tool cut marks: a carnivore kill followed by a human scavenger. Other bones bear the opposite: cut marks, then the marks of sharp teeth, saying there was a human with a weapon, then an animal with teeth. We come from a long line of hunters: 150,000 generations.[2]

This is what our line learned, and in the learning, we became human. We made tools to take what the grasses offered: large animals laden with nutrients, more nutrients than we could ever hope to find in fruit and leaves. The result is reading these words. Our brains are twice as large as they should be for a primate our size. Meanwhile our digestive tracts are 60 percent smaller. Our bodies were built by nutrient-dense foods. Anthropologists L. Aiello and P. Wheeler named this idea "The Expensive Tissue Hypothesis." The Australopithecine brain grew to Homo proportions because meat let our digestive systems shrink, thus freeing up energy for those brains.[3]

Or compare humans to gorillas. Gorillas are vegetarians and they have both the smallest brains and the largest digestive tracts of any primate. We are the opposite. And our brains, the true legacy of our ancestors, need to be fed.

The vegetarians have their own story, a very different one than the one told in the bones and tools, teeth and skulls. "Real strength and building material comes from green-leafed vegetables where the amino acids are found," writes one vegan guru. "If we look at the gorilla, zebra, giraffe, hippo, rhino, or elephant we find they build their enormous musculature on green-leafy vegetation."[4] Actually, if we really look at gorillas et al., what we find are animals that contain the fermentative bacteria necessary to digest cellulose. We humans contain no such thing. This man writes books about diet without knowing a thing about how humans actually digest.

For most of us, the bodies beneath our skin, inside our ribs, are unknown territory. But if we lay aside the story we long for and listen to our bodies, our biology will not lie. Here, then, is the long history that trees and savanna, grass and herds, have told in human tissue. (See table on following pages.)

There are two small differences between humans and dogs. One is that our canine teeth are shorter. The consensus is that ours were once longer than they currently are, but that they shrank due to our use of fire and tools. The other difference is that our intestines are longer, though clearly nowhere near as long as a sheep's. This is the remnant of our distant history as tree-dwelling fruitivores. And it's what grants us omnivorous status. But the chart on the following page should make clear what political and emotional attachments—and the FDA food pyramid—have obscured: we are built to consume meat, for the protein and fat it provides. Write Drs. Michael and Mary Dan Eades, "In anthropological scientific circles, there's absolutely no debate about it—every respected authority will confirm that we were hunters.... Our meat-eating heritage ... is an inescapable fact."[5]

There is another version of the story as well, one written by humans, not bones and teeth. This version lay waiting 40,000 years in caves from South Africa across Eurasia, and it's told in pictures. Some are schematics, the bare outlines of what matters. Others are lush with

	Human	**Dog**	**Sheep**
Teeth			
Incisors	Both Jaws	Both Jaws	Lower Jaw only
Molars	Ridged	Ridged	Flat
Canines	Small	Large	Absent
Jaw			
Movements	Vertical	Vertical	Rotary
Function	Tearing-Crushing	Tearing-Crushing	Grinding
Mastication	Unimportant	Unimportant	Vital Function
Rumination	Never	Never	Vital Function
Stomach			
Capacity	2 Quarts	2 Quarts	8.5 gallons
Emptying Time	3 Hours	3 Hours	Never Empties
Interdigestive Rest	Yes	Yes	No
Bacteria Present	No	No	Yes-Vital
Protozoa Present	No	No	Yes-Vital
Gastric Acidity	Strong	Strong	Weak
Cellulose Digestion	None	None	70%-Vital
Digestive Activity	Weak	Weak	Vital Function
Food Absorbed From	No	No	Vital Function
Gall Bladder			
Size	Well Developed	Well Developed	Often Absent
Function	Strong	Strong	Weak or Absent
Digestive Activity			
From Pancreas	Solely	Solely	Partial
From Bacteria	None	None	Partial
From Protozoa	None	None	Partial
Digestive Efficiency	100%	100%	50% or less

	Human	**Dog**	**Sheep**
Colon & Cecum			
Size of Colon	Short-Small	Short-Small	Long-Capacious
Size of Cecum	Tiny	Tiny	Long-Capacious
Function of Cecum	None	None	Vital Function
Appendix	Vestigial	Absent	Cecum
Rectum	Small	Small	Capacious
Digestive Activity	None	None	Vital Function
Cellulose Digestion	None	None	30%-Vital
Bacterial Flora	Putrefactive	Putrefactive	Fermentative
Food Absorbed From	None	None	Vital Function
Volume of Feces	Small-Firm	Small-Firm	Voluminous
Gross Food in Feces	Rare	Rare	Large Amount
Feeding Habits			
Frequency	Intermittent	Intermittent	Continuous
Survival Without			
Stomach	Possible	Possible	Impossible
Colon and Cecum	Possible	Possible	Impossible
Microorganisms	Possible	Possible	Impossible
Plant Foods	Possible	Possible	Impossible
Animal Protein	Impossible	Impossible	Possible
Ratio of Body Length to:			
Entire Digestive Tract	1:5	1:7	1:27
Small Intestine	1:4	1:6	1:25

Table from Walter L. Voegtlin's *The Stone Age Diet.*

texture and detail, the elements arranged so that the curves of the walls supply dimension and motion. "These bison," writes one observer, "seem to leap from a corner of the cave."[6] Or, as Pablo Picasso said on viewing the cave art of Lascaux, "We have invented nothing in twelve thousand years." No, we haven't. And even 40,000 years ago, it wasn't just us. The wild herds of aurochs and horses invented us out of their bodies, their nutrient-dense tissues gestating the human brain.

Some writers want to argue that hunting was the first act of domination, of political oppression. Yet life is only possible through death. Everything is dependent on killing, either directly or indirectly: you're either doing it or waiting for someone else to do it for you. Animals from praying mantids to bears hunt, and have you seen a kudzu vine take down a tree? Yet none of them, animal or vegetable, set up CAFOs or concentration camps. And though the human species must also kill, plenty of cultures have been built around reciprocity, humility, and basic kindness. If the getting of food, of life, means we are destined for sadism and genocide, then the universe is a sick and twisted place and I want out. But I don't believe it. It hasn't been my experience of food, of killing, of participating. When I see the art that people who were our anatomical equals made, I don't see a celebration of cruelty, an aesthetic of sadism. No, I wasn't there when the drawings were made and I didn't interview the artists. But I know beauty when I see it.

And the artists left no question about what they were eating. Besides their drawings, they also left weapons, including blades for killing and butchering. The tools are exquisite in their precision—and the ones made of wood are the oldest wooden objects ever found.

Archaeologists have dated an almost sixteen-inch-long spear tip carved of yew wood, found in 1911 in Clacton, England, to be somewhere between 360,000 and 420,000 years old. Another spear, also made of yew, is almost eight feet long and is 120,000 years old. It was found amid the ribs of an extinct elephant in Lehringen, Germany, in 1948. Excavators in a coal mine near Schoninger, Germany, found three spruce wood spears shaped like modern javelins—the longest of which measured over seven feet—that proved to be 300,000 to 400,000 years old.[7]

And our ancestors knew how to use their tools. *Fairweather Eden* is the story of the archaeological excavation in Boxgrove, England, a site lush with extinct rhinoceroses and wild horses, mammoths and cave bears. These animals were dangerous, large and strong, and not without defenses: a cave bear had teeth that were three inches long and "the jaw strength to snap a man in two."[8] If we could have simply lived on foraged fruit, wouldn't we have? But our hunger gave us courage, enough that we grew skilled. The archaeologists at Boxgrove took flint tools and a fresh-killed deer to the local butcher and asked him to take it apart with the tools. Five hundred thousand years later, the modern cut marks were exactly the same as the ancient ones.[9] We have, indeed, invented nothing.

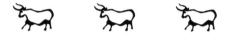

Except agriculture. And with agriculture comes the "diseases of civilization." Understand that no one speaks of the "diseases of hunter-gatherers," because they are largely disease-free. Not so the farmers, who have destroyed their bodies along with the planet. The list of diseases includes "[a]rthritis, diabetes, hypertension, heart disease, stroke, depression, schizophrenia, and cancer," as well as crooked teeth, bad eyesight, and a whole host of autoimmune and inflammatory conditions.[10]

These diseases are ubiquitous amongst the civilized and "are absolute rarities" for hunter-gatherers.[11] Writes Dr. Loren Cordain, in his article "Cereal Grains: Humanity's Double-Edged Sword":

> Cereal grains as a staple food are a relatively recent addition to the human diet and represent a dramatic departure from those foods to which we are genetically adapted. Discordance between humanity's genetically determined dietary needs and his [sic] present day diet is responsible for many of the degenerative diseases which plague industrial man.... [T]here is a significant body of evidence which suggests that cereal grains are less than optimal foods for humans and that the human

genetic makeup and physiology may not be fully adapted to high levels of cereal grain consumption.[12]

The archaeological evidence is incontrovertible, as is the living testament of the last extant eighty-four tribes of hunter-gatherers. They are eating the diet that all humans evolved to eat: "meat, fowl, fish and leaves, roots and fruits of many plants."[13] We are eating foods that didn't even exist until a few thousand years ago: domesticated annuals, especially grains, and even more their industrial endpoint of refined flours, sugars, and oils. As Cordain points out, "More than 70% of our dietary calories come from foods that our Paleolithic ancestors rarely, if ever, ate."[14] Our own bodies, with their degenerative diseases and overgrowth of cells, are all the evidence we need that this diet is unnatural.

So this is how we know what our ancestors ate: our teeth are made for meat, not cellulose; our stomachs are singular and secrete acid; both the tooth enamel and the art of our ancestors say so; human butchering tools are found beside butchered bones; and, to state the obvious, contemporary hunter-gatherers hunt.

One version of the vegetarian myth posits that we were "gatherer-hunters," gaining more sustenance from plants gathered by women than from meat hunted by men. This rumor actually has an author, one R.B. Lee, who concluded that hunter-gatherers got 65 percent of their calories from plants and only 35 percent from animals. This 65:35 figure has been repeated endlessly across disciplines, and it simply isn't true. Dr. Cordain ran a computer model with the plant foods accessible to hunter-gatherers. To meet their caloric needs alone, the 65:35 ratio would require eating twelve pounds of vegetation every day. "[A]n unlikely scenario, to say the least," comment the Drs. Eades.[15] Lee got his data from Murdock's *Ethnographic Atlas*, a collection of statistics from 862 different cultures. Of the 181 hunter-gatherer societies, Lee included only fifty-eight. He didn't count fish in his numbers, and he put shellfish in the "gathering" column. Tell me, have you ever been in danger of mistaking a lobster for a wild berry? The *Ethnographic Atlas* also classifies small land fauna—insects, grubs, reptiles, small mammals—as plants, by describing their collection as gathering. Cordain refigured the numbers as best he could, by reclassifying fish and shellfish as hunting, and by using data for all the available hunter-gatherers. His conclusion completely reversed Lee's numbers. He suggests that the true ratio is closer to 65 percent animal to 35 percent plants. And that's still including the *Ethnographic Atlas*'s bias of small land fauna as plants.[16]

The first myth of the nutritional vegetarians—that we aren't meant for meat—is another fairy tale filled with inedible apples. I try to remember what I believed when I was a vegan. There was a mythic golden age, long ago, when we lived in harmony with the world ... and ... ate what? Prehistoric paintings of humans hunting left me confused and defensive, but I was unclear on the timeline anyway. Maybe all that hunting happened before the peaceful vegetarian Goddess culture? Or maybe it was *after* the fall of the peaceful vegetarian ...?

We ate grains, I decided, and a lot of unnamed leafy things. Never mind that grains were "not even in existence for the majority of our time on earth."[17] Or that they would not have been available more than one month out of twelve. Or that the technologies needed to make them edible weren't invented until the birth of agriculture. Grains have to be ground, soaked, and most of all, cooked. You can't eat wheat raw. Try it if you don't believe me, but you don't have to: you will get sick with gastroenteritis. This is true for grains, beans, and potatoes. They contain toxins, politely known as anti-nutrients, to stop animals (us) from eating them. Just because plants can't scream and run doesn't mean they want to be eaten. And just because they don't have teeth or claws doesn't mean they aren't fighting back. Heat is what makes them edible by disabling some of the antinutrients. Grinding, soaking, rinsing, and sprouting also help. But understand the lengths to which plants have gone to protect themselves and their precious offspring, their biological future, and what we have done to ourselves by eating them.

First, plants produce enzyme blockers, which act as a pesticide against insects and other animals, including us. Our digestive systems utilize many enzymes to break down and absorb food. When the food is seeds (beans, grains, potatoes), the seeds resist by blocking those enzymes. The most common enzymes that grains try to disrupt are proteases, which digest protein. Proteases include the stomach enzyme pepsin and the small intestine enzymes trypsin and chymotrypsin. Other chemicals interfere with amylase, the enzyme that digests starch, and hence are called amylase inhibitors.

Beans, grains, and potatoes also use lectins, which are proteins that fill a huge variety of functions in both plants and animals, though the exact function of many lectins is still unknown. In order to understand the damage that these substances can do to the human body, you first need a basic primer on human digestion.

Our digestive tract has a tough job: it has to sort through a huge array of foreign substances—the things we swallow—and decide what's a nutrient and what's a danger. The ones deemed nutrients have to be broken down into the smallest possible components and then absorbed. This work is so labor intensive that your intestines measure twenty-two feet. To increase the work capacity, the intestines are folded up into compacted gathers called villi. "In fact," explain the Drs. Eades, "the folds are so tightly packed that if you were to flatten them into a sheet, a single centimeter (less than half an inch) of intestinal lining would cover a doubles tennis court—an astounding bit of origami."[18]

Microvilli are even smaller folds. They comprise what's called the brush border, the area where digestive enzymes break proteins down into their constituent amino acids and starches down into sugars. Once food is completely broken down, the lining of the gut lets nutrients into the bloodstream through what are called tight junctions. These are specialized seals between the lining cells. We need to be protected from all sorts of contaminants and toxins that travel from the outside world, past our teeth, and through our stomachs. The tight junctions are the place where substances are either absorbed or rejected. Too big, too scary, or too foreign and they can't get through the tight junctions. But anything small and simple—water, ions, amino acids, and sugars—gets a pass.

That's one mechanical way that our intestines keep us safe. Another is through the rhythmic contractions that keep the input moving through the intestines. The constant motion stops unfriendly bacteria from setting up residence. And the lining cells are continuously shedding, so any bacteria that have managed to grab a hold of our guts are carried away.

If these mechanical methods fail, our guts can also mount an immunological defense, and it's a very specialized defense. The usual immune response elsewhere in the body involves inflammation. Not so in the gut, and if you can picture the surface area of a tennis court folding itself into half a square inch you'll see why. There's no room for inflammation, not if that area wants to absorb nutrients, too. Inflammation would weaken the tight junctions, rendering us vulnerable to dangerous substances that could slip into our bodies. Instead, the gut operates its own rapid response team. Specialized cells take any invaders prisoner. Another set of cells, lymphocytes, will start manufacturing poisons to kill the invading substances. "And not only that," write the Drs. Eades, "the armed lymphocytes will remember the face of the invader forever, so that if one like it ever cares to show up again, the immune response will be swift and sure."[19]

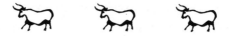

Eating grains causes three problems. The first is that a grain-based diet will include too many starches and sugars, which will overload the intestines. The gut in turn will pass them on undigested to the colon. These sugars create "a veritable bacterial picnic," and the colon's normal population of bacteria experiences exponential growth.[20] This over-productive fermentation can then surge back into the gut, causing an inflammatory response which "blunts its bristly microvilli, impairs proper digestion and absorption, and, in the beginnings of a vicious cycle, sends even more incompletely digested foods downstream."[21] Most crucially, the tight junctions are damaged, letting substances like lectins pass through into the bloodstream. And the lectins themselves may bind to the wall of the intestines, altering their permeability and their function.

So what are lectins? Krispin Sullivan explains:

> Think of a lectin as a protein containing a key that fits a
> certain type of lock. This lock is a specific type of carbohy-
> drate.... If a lectin with the right key comes in contact with
> one of these 'locks' on the gut wall or artery or gland or or-
> gan, it 'opens the lock', that is, it disrupts the membrane and
> damages the cell and may initiate a cascade of immune and
> autoimmune events leading to cell death.[22]

Lectins don't break down without a fight: once they're ingested, neither hydrochloric acid nor digestive enzymes can destroy them. In fact, "WGA [wheat germ agglutinin, a cereal grain lectin] is heat stable and resistant to digestive proteolytic breakdown in both rats and humans and has been recovered intact and biologically active in human feces."[23] Over 60 percent of lectins "remain ... immunologically intact" in the digestive tract.[24] Because of this, the damage they can do is immense.

By the time a meal clears the stomach and enters the intestines, any protein we've eaten should have been broken down into amino acids. This helps keep larger components from passing through the wall of the intestines and into the bloodstream. Smaller bits do sometimes make it through, but the amounts aren't enough to trigger an immune response. But because lectins are able to survive the human stomach intact, the "concentrations of lectins can be quite high, consequently their transport through the gut wall can exceed that of other dietary antigens by several orders of magnitude."[25]

Lectins can also bond to the walls of the intestines and damage their permeability. Their bonding creates everything from shortened villi to changes in intestinal flora to cell death. This combination of sheer concentration of lectins and damaged guts means that lectins pass through the intestines whole. Once they get past that basic defensive barrier, they wreak havoc all over the human body.

The profound destruction that lectins are capable of lies in the autoimmune response they can trigger. The protein sequence in some lectins is almost identical to tissues in the human body.[26] Once the lectins pass through the compromised tight junctions and into the bloodstream, they cause tremendous and tragic damage in a process called *molecular mimicry*. The immune defense system attacks the foreign proteins, and having learned to identify that sequence as an enemy, it goes on to attack the similar sequences in the human body. The lectin in wheat is made of amino acid sequences that mimic both joint cartilage and the myelin sheaths that cover our nerves. [27] Other lectins are nearly identical to the filtering mechanism of the kidneys, the cells of the pancreas that produce insulin, the retina, the lining of our intestines. And once turned on, the immune system doesn't turn off. Lectins confuse the immune system, teaching it that some primary parts of "us" are a "them." The lesson learned becomes the terrible suffering of a body attacking itself, the autoimmune diseases such as "Crohn's disease ... ulcerative colitis, rheumatoid arthritis, ankylosing spondylitis, systemic lupus erythematosus, psoriasis, type 1 diabetes mellitus, glomerulonephritis ... multiple sclerosis, and potentially many others as well—from thyroid inflammation to allergies to skin rashes to asthma."[28]

The molecular mimicry of lectins may not be the only catalyst for autoimmune diseases. Some researchers are also investigating viruses and bacteria. For instance, the bacteria *M. paratuberculosis*, which causes Johne's disease in ruminants, may be implicated in Crohn's disease in humans. There may be multiple causes for autoimmune diseases or there may be a precipitating load of foreign substances that triggers an autoimmune cascade.

But epidemiologists do know that multiple sclerosis—an autoimmune disease where the body attacks its own nerve sheaths—is most prevalent in cultures where wheat and rye are staple foods. In the archaeological record, rheumatoid arthritis, which leaves very grim evidence in skeletal remains, follows wheat and corn around the world.[29] Celiac disease is absolutely caused by cereal grains, and celiac sufferers are at risk for other autoimmune diseases. They are also *thirty times* more likely to be schizophrenic. In fact, numerous clinical studies show that removing gluten from the diet ameliorates schizophrenia.[30]

Yet it wasn't until 1950 that a Dutch pediatrician, Dr. Willem Dicke, made the connection between wheat and celiac disease. "Indeed," writes Cordain, "it is astounding that humanity was unaware, until only relatively recently, that an ordinary and commonplace food such as cereal grains could be responsible for a disease which afflicts between 1 and 3.5 people per 1,000 in Europe."[31]

I actually don't think it's astounding. I think it's almost impossible for most people to step outside their culture and question its practices, especially those practices where power and taboo coalesce—sex, religion, food. To understand that agricultural foods are not the foods we were designed to eat throws the entire project of civilization into a new and uneasy light, and who is willing to do that?

Yet the truth about agriculture is there, waiting in the wreckage of our bodies like it waits in the broken skeletons of forests and in exsanguinated wetlands. Paleopathologists tell us that "autoimmune disorders do not seem to have plagued humans prior to the adoption of an agricultural way of life."[32] That's because it's grains that can turn the body against itself. Agriculture has devoured us as surely as it has devoured the world.

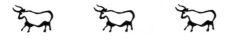

And just as agriculture has displaced species-dense communities with its monocrops, its diet has displaced the nutrient-dense foods that humans need, replacing them with mononutrients of sugar and starch. This displacement led immediately to a drop in human stature as agriculture spread—the evidence couldn't be clearer. The reasons are just as clear. Meat contains protein, minerals, and fats, fats that we need to metabolize those proteins and minerals. In contrast, grains are basically carbohydrates: what protein they do contain is low quality—lacking essential amino acids—and comes wrapped in indigestible fiber. Grains are essentially sugar with enough opioids to make them addictive.

The biological truth will be hard to face if, like me, you built the entire superstructure of your identity on a foundation of grain. But these are the facts. There are essential amino acids, the so-called building blocks of protein. They're essential because humans can't make them; we can only eat them. Likewise, there are essential fatty acids—fats—which, despite being vilified, can only be ingested, not made.

And carbohydrates? There is no such thing as a necessary carbo-hydrate. Read that again. Write the Drs. Eades, "the actual amount of carbohydrates *required* by humans for health is *zero*."[33]

Every cell in your body can make all the sugar it needs. That in-cludes the cells in your hungry brain. The detractors of low-carb diets have created and endlessly repeated the myth that our brains need glucose and hence we need to eat carbohydrates. Yes, our brains do need glucose—which is precisely why our bodies can *make* glucose. What the brain actually needs is a very steady supply of glucose: too much or too little will create a biological emergency that can result in coma and death, as any diabetic will tell you. And a constant cycle of too much/too little is exactly what a carbohydrate-based diet will pro-vide, leaving a wreckage of deteriorating organs and arteries behind. A partial list of diseases caused by high insulin levels includes "heart disease, elevated cholesterol, elevated triglycerides, high blood pres-sure, blood clotting problems, colon cancer (and a number of other cancers), type II diabetes, gout, sleep apnea, obesity, iron-overload disease, gastroesophageal reflux (severe heartburn), peptic ulcer dis-ease, [and] polycystic ovary disease."[34]

These are serious diseases and they are endemic to civilized cultures. We accept them as normal because they are ubiquitous. We eat the foods our culture provides; we get sick. But then everyone is sick—who doesn't know someone with diabetes, cancer, heart disease, arthritis?—so no one questions it. And it's a lot to question, from the USDA food pyramid, to the righteous aura with which the Left has infused plant-based foods, to civilization itself. These are power-ful forces to which our own native intelligence—both personal and cultural—has long been subordinated.

What we are left with are cravings, both vague and unbearable, that we have taught ourselves to fight. "When I eat, I feel full," a friend of mine said. "But when I eat at your house, I feel nourished." Believe me, it's not my skill as a chef she's acknowledging. It's the quality of the ingredients: real food. Real protein and real fats from animals who in turn ate *their* real food.

"I've never had anything like this," another visitor stammered in awe, after her first bite of *crème brûlée*. It's a reaction I've gotten used to. She'd never had eggs from chickens who happily lounged and hunted and lounged some more in woods and pastures, nor cream from heirloom cows who spent contented lives with their heads in the grass. Those details matter, not just morally and politically, but also nutritionally, which we will return to later. My point here is that our bodies still respond to the food we were meant for, even if we've never had it, even if we think we shouldn't have it. The *crème brûlée* enthusiast's diet consisted of mostly wheat and rice, with a few eggs from caged, tormented, and misfed hens, some anemic sugar-laced yogurt scoured of fat, and industrially manufactured soy products. Do I need to add that she was intensely hypoglycemic and had early osteoporosis? Listen to your hunger, was how I wanted to answer her, instead of with the slow explanation of grass and fats, animals and us, life and death, that I had to give.

Listen to your body, reader, a listening that must make your body known to you, less mysterious and more beloved. The listening is hard. You will have to hear past the propaganda of the agriculturalists, both the corrupt and the righteous. You will also have to listen past the cravings that those foods produce: the addictions to opioids and intense sweeteners, the biological emergencies of blood sugar swings. And you will have to accept "the soft animal of your body," as poet Mary Oliver so sweetly says, not punish it.[35]

These are daunting obstacles, and if you can't find your way clear to the true hunger beneath, maybe the damage of a plant-based diet can lead you there. Maybe you don't find the molecular mimicry of autoimmune disorders strong enough evidence. Then listen to this instead: "The diseases that insulin affects directly ... are the cause of the vast majority of death and disability in the US today. They are the grim reapers of Western civilization."[36] Heart disease, high blood pressure, and diabetes are all caused by the insulin surges that grain and sugar demand.

What's the difference between complex carbohydrates and sugar? Despite the intense propaganda to declare the former "good" and the latter "bad," not much. "Many people are of the opinion that there are good and bad carbohydrates, when in actuality there are barely tolerable and awful sugars," write the Drs. Eades.[37] Whether "complex" or "simple," all carbohydrates are sugars. The only difference is whether they are individual sugar molecules or a string of sugar molecules. Glucose is the simplest sugar, made of a single molecule. Sucrose, regular table sugar, is made of two molecules and is, hence, a disaccharide. There are three-molecule trisaccharides. Sugars with more molecules are called polysaccharides. These include grains, beans, and potatoes.

Why don't these differences matter? Because our digestive system can't digest the long chains. They're too big to be absorbed through the intestinal wall. So our bodies break them down into simple sugars. And every last molecule eventually hits the bloodstream:

> So whether it began life as a fat-free bagel, a quarter cup of sugar from the sugar bowl, a canned soft drink, a bowl of fettuccine, a baked potato, or a handful of jelly beans, by the time your intestinal tract gets finished snipping the links of those starch and sugar chains, it's all been reduced to ... sugar. Specifically, to glucose. And in the end there's very little metabolic difference between your eating a medium baked potato or drinking a 12-ounce can of soda pop. Each contains about fifty grams of easily digestible and rapidly available glucose. It may surprise you to know that the potato might even be slightly worse in terms of the rise in blood sugar that follows it.[38]

According to the USDA, we should be eating a diet that is 60 percent carbohydrate. Your body will turn that carbohydrate into almost *two cups* of glucose, and each and every molecule has to be reckoned with.

That amount of sugar in the bloodstream would lead to coma and death if humans didn't have a way to process sugar, and fast. So the body comes equipped with a mechanism to clear sugar from the blood, but it's a mechanism that agriculturalists wear out. Elevated sugar levels stimulate the pancreas to produce insulin. Insulin is a hormone responsible for nutrient storage. Its primary purpose is to get excess sugar, amino acids, and fats out of the blood and into the cells.

Sugar is the most dangerous of those three, as too much sugar can cause serious consequences very quickly. So insulin's most important job is to keep blood sugar levels out of the red zone. It does this by binding with insulin receptors, which are proteins on a cell's surface that remove sugar from the blood. Insulin is the switch that turns on the insulin receptors, which then do the work of moving glucose into the cell.

Patients with juvenile diabetes have pancreases that produce very little insulin. Their insulin receptors are in working order, but without the stimulating presence of insulin, their receptors are never triggered to act. That's why these patients take insulin.

Type II diabetes has a different etiology. Eating any carbohydrate or sugar results in a glucose surge in the bloodstream. The pancreas responds with insulin, insulin triggers the insulin receptors, and the insulin receptors pump sugar into the cells for immediate use or for storage. So far, so good.

The problem comes with overuse. When blood sugar levels are constantly spiking from a diet high in carbohydrates, the amount of insulin required to deal with that will, over time, damage the insulin receptors, blunting their ability to work. Yet the high levels of sugar still need to be lowered, and lowered quickly. So the pancreas pumps out even more insulin, which temporarily forces the insulin receptors into action but ultimately creates still more damage. Now there is so much insulin in the blood that by the time it's all bound to the insulin receptors, blood sugar levels will be too low. This cycle, of high blood sugar → too much insulin → low blood sugar, is called hypoglycemia, and it ends when the sufferer, biologically desperate to raise her blood sugar levels, puts another dose of sugar into her mouth with a sweaty, shaking hand. That will help, for an hour or two—until her blood sugar crashes again and the whole process starts over.

Where it really ends is in type II diabetes. The resistant insulin receptors demand too much insulin, more than the pancreas could ever make. The chronic excess sugar destroys the nerves, the arteries, the retinas, the heart. Despite every advance in medical science, a diabetic's life can be shortened by one third.[39] Such are the wages of civilization's dietary sins.

Because insulin also controls a number of other basic life functions, high levels of insulin will cause damage throughout the body. Insulin triggers cholesterol synthesis, activating the enzymes that spur cholesterol production. About 85 percent of your cholesterol is made in your body: only 15 percent is dietary, which is one reason why low-fat diets have proven basically useless. Though every one of your cells both makes and needs cholesterol, most of it is produced in the liver. Elevated insulin means elevated cholesterol. The Drs. Eades explain why.

> Excess food energy increases blood sugar, which increases insulin, which triggers the storage cycle leading to fat accumulation. To store fat and build muscle, the body must make new cells, and insulin acts as a growth hormone for this process. Cholesterol plays a vital role in this building and storing process; cholesterol provides the structural framework for all cells.[40]

And high blood pressure, heart disease, and arteriosclerosis? Too much insulin triggers the growth of smooth muscle cells that line the arteries, thickening the walls and reducing elasticity. Blood volume of the arteries shrinks, which means the heart has to pump harder, which is another way of saying "high blood pressure." Insulin also triggers the kidneys to retain fluid, which again increases blood pressure. Arteries with less elasticity are more prone to plaquing and arterial spasm, which are the causes of heart disease. Insulin also encourages fibrous connective tissue to grow inside the arteries, providing a scaffold for the first layer of plaque.

Insulin increases oxidation of LDL particles. These hard-working substances have been declared guilty for no good reason and dubbed "bad cholesterol." Like the rest of us, they're only bad when they're damaged. And what damages them? Too much blood sugar and insulin. Sugars are able to attach to proteins all over the body and start a reaction that creates permanent damage to the cells. This process is called glycation and fructation, for glucose and fructose, respectively. It's similar to how "dairy protein and fat with sugar and heat ... make caramel."[41] The Drs. Eades explain:

Year in and year out, from the time we're born, this damage wrought by the carmelization process accumulates in our bodies; over a lifetime it wreaks the most havoc in long-lived proteins, including elastin, the protein that gives youthful elasticity to the skin; crystallin, the special protein that forms the lens of the eye; DNA, the genetic blueprint present in all cells; and collagen, the structural protein that accounts for over 30 percent of the body's protein mass, occurring in tissues all over the body, including the hair, skin, and nails, the walls of all arteries and veins, and the framework of bones and organs. Damage to these critical protein structures results not only in such cosmetic maladies as wrinkles and age spots, but in serious health problems ranging from cataracts to failure of major organs, such as the kidneys and the heart.[42]

That's just from ingesting sugar. The excess insulin required by that ingestion makes it even worse: insulin raises the rate of oxidation of the LDL particles. So on a carbohydrate-based diet, there's lots of sugar to do damage, and that sugar requires insulin that adds even more damage. Once impaired, the LDL heads for the arterial walls. There, it sets off an immune reaction. The body's defenders, the macrophages, will attack and dismember the LDL, creating inflammation and vanquished bits of deranged cholesterol. Those bits are now bioavailable and will be used by the body in the formation of plaque.

Insulin triggers the production of fibrinogen, which is the substance used in the first stage of clot formation. Insulin also stimulates the kidneys to dump both magnesium and potassium, which can lead to heart arrhythmias and life-threatening fibrillation. Is there any stage of coronary heart disease missing from this indictment?

The counterbalancing hormone to insulin is glucagon. When your blood sugar levels are in free fall and headed for the crash, glucagon's job is to get those levels back up. It does this by stimulating the body to burn its reserves of energy, and it has some help: both adrenaline and cortisol are part of the process. Remember that a blood sugar level out of a narrow range—either too low or too high—is a life-threatening emergency, and it requires emergency measures. Adrenaline prepares you for fight or flight. It forces energy out of storage and cranks up the metabolism in your muscles, getting you ready for action. One of the ways it frees up more energy for your muscles is by shutting down your digestive systems: the presence of adrenaline suppresses the stomach's production of hydrochloric acid.

That's fine for the occasional sabertooth tiger attack, but eating a high-carbohydrate diet is a tiger attack three times a day, every day. You can damage your stomach's ability to produce hydrochloric acid, and anyone with blood sugar problems is at risk. The resulting condition is called gastroparesis, and I gave it to myself. Writes Dr. Tom Cowan:

> One of the clues to healing gastroparesis is the fact that it most commonly occurs in those who are either diabetic or who have hypothyroidism. Blood sugar regulation is intimately tied to the functioning of the stomach and the health of the nerves. Very low-carbohydrate diets have been successfully used in virtually all stomach disorders because it has been found that insulin is intimately tied up with acid production, the pressure at the esophageal-gastric sphincter and the hormonal control of other stomach functions. Lowering insulin levels through a low carbohydrate diet ... is the first step in resolving this disorder.[43]

For fourteen years I felt sick, nauseated, and bloated. Anything I ate became a bowling ball lodged in my stomach. When I say fourteen years, I mean fourteen years solid. The only time it subsided was if I didn't eat for forty-eight hours. No doctor ever diagnosed it correctly or helped—until I found a doctor who worked with recovering vegans. Three weeks on betaine hydrochloride, a form of hydrochloric acid, and the nausea was gone. Am I allowed to call it a miracle? I know that on the scale of global horrors my stomach ranks as the tiniest nanoblip, but it's my nanoblip, and that constant bloated nausea was awful.

So here are some questions for you, vegetarians. Do you feel sick when you eat? Specifically, does your stomach feel distended, bloated, or like it takes a long time to empty? It's not your blood type and it's not because you're "naturally" meant to "eat light"—two things I've heard a lot from vegetarians afflicted with mysterious stomach ailments. If you can't eat the food your body needs, it's because you've damaged your digestion, from too many blood sugar highs and lows, and too much adrenaline. It can be fixed, but you're going to have to eat real protein and fat and not sugars. You need to leave adrenaline for emergencies only: can we agree that breakfast shouldn't be one?

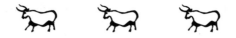

Cholesterol is, of course, the bulwark that the nutritional vegetarians will stand behind. The Lipid Hypothesis—the theory that ingested fat causes heart disease—is the stone tablet that the Prophets of Nutrition have brought down from the mountain. We have been shown the one, true way: cholesterol is the demon of the age, the dietary Black Plague, a judgment from an angry God, condemning those who stray into the Valley of Animal Products with disease. That at least is what the priests of the Lipid Hypothesis declared, having looked into the entrails of ... rabbits.

Rabbits?

Yes, it all began when researchers fed protein and cholesterol to rabbits and their blood cholesterol shot up. And it reached numbers never seen in humans. The cholesterol was in the rabbits' arteries, but it produced a different kind of lesion than in humans, and the animals never developed advanced plaques in their blood vessels. Instead, cholesterol accumulated in their organs, resulting in fatty buildup in their kidneys and livers, discolored eyes, and loss of fur. These force-fed rabbits didn't die from coronary disease; they died from starvation because they lost their appetites. Which is about what you'd expect when you take an herbivore designed for cellulose and stuff her full of fat and protein.

This haruspicy has also been done on "chickens, guinea pigs, pigeons, parrots, goats, rats and mice" with similar arterial deposits developing.[44]

When these experiments are done on carnivores—cats, dogs, foxes—no damage results. In dogs, cholesterol feeding had no effect at all unless the poor creatures had their thyroids removed or chemically suppressed.[45]

Writes Anthony Colpo, "High amounts of cholesterol appeared to be readily metabolized by carnivorous animals, whereas herbivorous animals may not be equipped to metabolize large amounts of dietary cholesterol or animal fat, both of which are absent from plant foods."[46]

Not to put too fine a point on it, but duh?

Remember that 80 percent of the cholesterol in your blood was made by your body. Only 20 percent was put there by your food choices. Your body knows where it wants that cholesterol level. It may have been misled—by insulin, for instance—but it will adjust its production based on what you ingest. If you eat more cholesterol, it will produce less. A meta-analysis of *one hundred sixty seven*—yes, that's 167—cholesterol-feeding experiments found that raising dietary cholesterol had a negligible effect on blood cholesterol, and no link to CHD (coronary heart disease) risk.[47]

Before we go any further, do you even know what cholesterol is? This benign, maligned substance is needed by every cell in your body, and most of all by the ones that make you human. Cholesterol is technically a sterol, not a fat. One of the main functions of the liver is to make cholesterol, not because your liver wants you dead, but because life isn't possible without cholesterol. Low levels of cholesterol may very well kill people. The increased mortality due to *low* cholesterol is serious enough that the National Heart, Lung and Blood Institute of the National Institutes of Health held a conference to explore researchers' findings on the subject.[48] "Evidence from a multitude of sources was presented linking low blood cholesterol levels to an increase in various cancers, hemorrhagic stroke, respiratory and digestive diseases, and violent death," Colpo sums up.[49] In France, a study of 6,000 men over seventeen years showed that those whose cholesterol declined the most had the *highest* risk for cancer.[50] Or how about the heart failure patients whose risk of death was twice as high for those with the *lowest* cholesterol levels?[51] There's a lot more, but none of it will make sense until you understand that cholesterol is a life-sustaining substance, not a murderer inside your blood.

Cholesterol has a special trick that plays a crucial role in animal bodies: it doesn't dissolve in water. Our internal environment is liquid. Hence, cell membranes need to be structurally stable. Without cholesterol, you would be a puddle, not an animal. Your cell membranes also need to be waterproof. This is especially true for the cells of your nervous system, including your brain, which is one reason why more cholesterol is found there than anywhere else.

Cholesterol is also the body's basic repair substance. The integrity of your intestinal wall especially depends on it. And cholesterol has antioxidant powers, keeping cancer-causing free radicals from doing their damage. Finally, all of your hormones, including your sex hormones, are made from cholesterol.

Does that sound so awful?

As a culture, we've been collectively sitting around the campfire and, while night takes hold, listening to the big kids like the American Heart Association and the USDA. They've been telling us a story about an escapee from a mental hospital with an alias of Cholesterol and a hook for a hand ... The grownups are there in the background, telling us it's not true, but when do we listen to them?

One of the big kids was Ancel Keys, who assembled the famous Six Countries Study. Figure 4A shows what he wanted you to know.

This "study" is absurd for two reasons. To understand them, you need the basic science education that the public school system failed to provide. The whole point of an experiment is to test a hypothesis. You do that by eliminating as many variables as possible. With epidemiological evidence like the Keys study, it's impossible. That's why epidemiological studies can only prove correlation. They cannot prove causality. They may suggest intriguing areas for exploration but until all the variables are controlled and the results are reproducible, no conclusions can be drawn. The kind of cross-country comparison that Keys did "involves comparing apples with oranges—that is countries with widely varying cultural, social, political and physical environments."[52] With such an infinite number of variables, a finding of definitive causation would be ridiculous.

John Yudkin's 1957 study shows the error of conflating correlation with causation. You can see from Figure 4B (page over) that

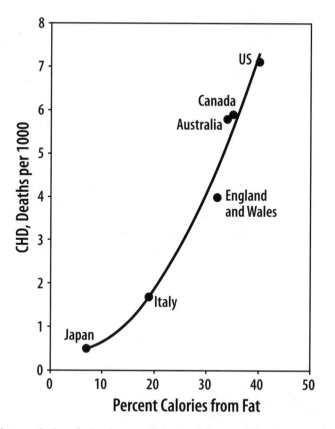

Figure 4A. Correlation between the total fat consumption as a percent of total calorie consumption, and mortality from coronary heart disease in six countries. Redrawn from *The Cholesterol Myths* by Uffe Ravnskov.

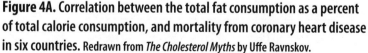

owning a TV and radio had a much stronger association with Coronary Heart Disease (CHD) than any nutritional elements.[53] But no one would suggest that TV causes CHD, or that sacrificing our TVs will grant us a longer life. No one went on to investigate whether TVs produced heart-stopping emissions or blood-damaging toxins. No government health agency paid for people to throw out their TVs as a treatment for CHD. No one mistook association for causation.

Dr. Uffe Ravnskov made a graph (Figure 4C, page over) showing that income tax rates correlate with CHD. According to his graph, if the tax rate dropped below 9.55 percent, the good citizens of Sweden would be free of the scourge of CHD.[54]

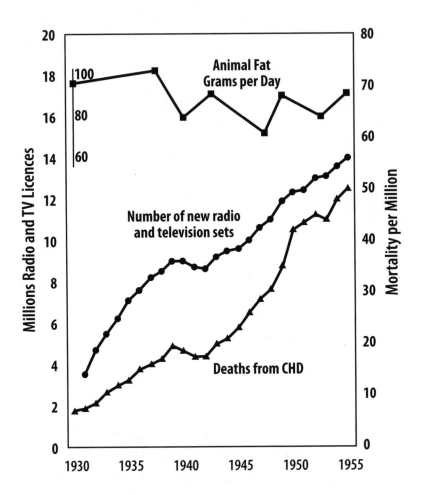

Figure 4B. Consumption of animal fat, number of new radio and television sets and number of deaths from coronary disease in England and Wales between 1910 and 1956. Redrawn from *The Cholesterol Myths* by Uffe Ravnskov.

These kinds of epidemiological studies make for snappy headlines. I see them all the time. There was one recently about body weight and sleep. Apparently researchers correlated subjects' weight and the amount they slept, and the relationship was an inverse proportion. The more you weigh, the less you sleep. Does that mean that if you sleep more you lose weight? To judge by the message boards, a fair number of people jumped right from correlation to causality, with

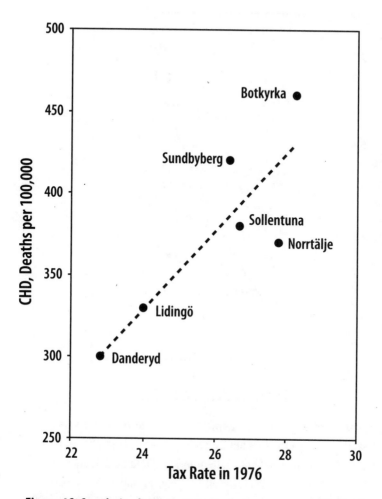

Figure 4C. Correlation between tax rate and coronary mortality in the municipal tax districts of the county of Stockholm, Sweden. According to this graph, if the tax rate drops to 9.55 percent, CHD will be conquered. Redrawn from *The Cholesterol Myths* by Uffe Ravnskov.

no stop in between at rationality. Yes, it's one possible explanation for the correlation: less sleep somehow causes weight gain. So more sleep might help you lose weight. It could just as easily be the other way around: more body weight causes insomnia, and sleeping more will only help the insomnia. Or it could be a million other things.

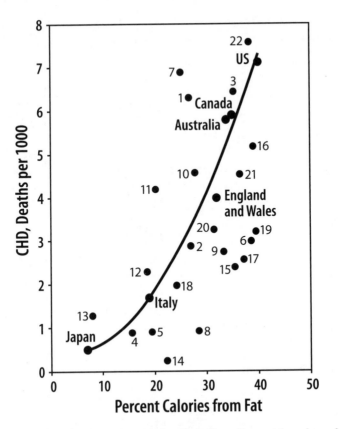

Figure 4D. Same as Figure 4A, but including all countries where data were available when Dr. Keys published his paper. 1. Australia; 2. Italy; 3. Canada; 4. Sri Lanka; 5. Chile; 6. Denmark; 7. Finland; 8. France; 9. West Germany; 10. Ireland; 11. Israel; 12. Italy; 13. Japan; 14. Mexico; 15. Holland; 16. New Zealand; 17. Norway; 18. Portugal; 19. Sweden; 20. Switzerland; 21. Great Britain; 22. USA. Redrawn from *The Cholesterol Myths* by Uffe Ravnskov.

My point here is to never, ever put your money—let alone your physical well-being—on an epidemiological study. And learn to distinguish between correlation and causality. Or, as one set of researchers put it, after their high-fat data refuted their low-fat hypothesis, "Observational studies on populations are only useful for formulating hypotheses and they cannot provide convincing evidence of cause-and-effect relations."[55]

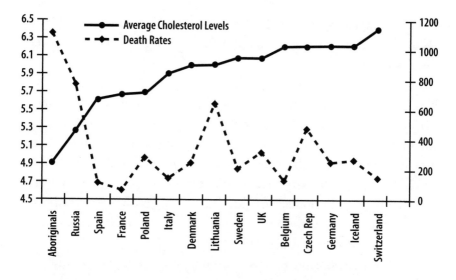

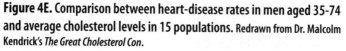

Figure 4E. Comparison between heart-disease rates in men aged 35-74 and average cholesterol levels in 15 populations. Redrawn from Dr. Malcolm Kendrick's *The Great Cholesterol Con*.

Keys only used numbers that supported his point. He had nutritional data from twenty-two countries and he only used the ones that he liked. Figure 4D restores all the data he excluded. You can see how his hypothesis is utterly refuted by the data that he had—and willfully ignored. Another researcher, Dr. George Mann, found that Keys had also removed those countries that correlated lack of exercise to CHD.[56] Even on its own terms, Keys' study was a disaster until he tortured the data.

Dr. Malcolm Kendrick put together a similar chart (see Figure 4E) using updated data from the MONICA project of the WHO (World Health Organization). MONICA stands for "MONitor trends in CArdiovascular diseases." It was the single largest investigation into diet and CHD *ever*, including nutritional data from twenty-one countries and ten million people over ten years.

The results? Not even a correlation between cholesterol levels, fat intake, and cardiovascular mortality.

Kendrick also notes that if Keys had chosen Germany, Switzerland, France, and Sweden instead of Greece, Former Yugoslavia,

USA, and Japan, Keys would have "shown" the opposite correlation, "Namely, the more saturated fat and cholesterol consumed the lower the risk of CHD." [57]

But the big kids over at the American Heart Association, the USDA, and Pfizer like their one-hooked villain. Though this information has been available for forty years, and numerous doctors and researchers have been decrying the Lipid Hypothesis as a fraud for as long, the orthodoxy still refers to "the Keys Equation" as "the most precise way to predict the effect of diet on the blood cholesterol levels of individuals and populations, and thus, their risk of coronary heart disease."[58] Clearly it's up to us to figure out the truth about diet and health, fats and hearts, cause and effect.

CHD is responsible for vast amounts of death and disability in the US. I hope the evidence presented so far—especially the visual evidence—is compelling, hopefully compelling enough to be liberatory. Throw out that sickly canola margarine, that inedible skim milk, those endless fat-free soy extrusions whose only flavor is a rancid aftertaste you've vowed to ignore. Your body—your brain, your bones, and your heart—is hungry, and somewhere inside you, you know it's true. You have nothing to lose but your punishment.

If you want to dig deeper into the research, if you need more information to feel like you're on solid ground before an undertaking as serious as a dietary overhaul, I suggest the following guidelines.

1. Epidemiological studies are of limited use, since the endless number of variables they include can't be controlled.

2. If you do look at epidemiological studies, take care never ever to conflate correlation with causality.

3. Controlled studies are a better bet, but read them carefully. Do not ever believe the headline sound bite on Yahoo! News. And don't just trust the conclusions, but read the whole study. Data is often starved or force-fed to support the bias of the researcher. See for yourself whether every variable was the same *except for the one being*

tested. And follow the money. Be ultra-wary of studies funded by drug manufacturers.

4. Never trust just one study, no matter how good it looks or how much you like its conclusions. Remember the basic principle of science: the results have to be reproducible to count.

5. Heed the words of Jessica Prentice, author of *Full Moon Feast*, who writes, "Although bookstores are full of advice on how to be healthy or thin, or both, and there is a constant stream of media telling us which foods are good for us and which bad, I have found very little of what I hear about food in contemporary America to be useful to me. The surfeit of information doesn't help me eat well—in fact, it confuses me and sets me back."[59]

I've been through that same confusion, which can feel as strong as terror, when something as basic as food, and as primary as identity, gives way, and the stable rules of good and bad, me and not me, collapse. You may feel driven to shore up those rules after viewing some of the graphs presented here. I have known that impulse, sometimes desperately, and it's a very human reaction. But to pursue the truth, we have to leave room for the possibility that we might be ignorant, or even wrong. We have to accept confusion, embrace the risk of not knowing. As a culture we've lost the moorings of traditional lifeways and their foods. Corporate America began taking over the food stream in the 1920s, and the process has been complete for over a generation. We have very little to go on, and the experts our culture offers in the place of wisdom have not proven trustworthy. If we acknowledge that this is difficult—that we are in for a bit of Mr. Toad's Wild Ride—it will go easier.

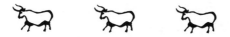

In order for the Lipid Hypothesis to become the Lipid Law, the following dots would have to be connected. Saturated fat would have to raise cholesterol levels, and cholesterol would have to cause CHD.

Saturated fat → raised cholesterol → CHD

There is a huge array of epidemiological studies that show no
correlation between saturated fat consumption, cholesterol levels,
and heart disease. Let's look at some of those first, not because I
think they're so great as a concept, but because proponents of the
Lipid Hypothesis love epidemiological studies so much. First are all
the paradoxes: the French Paradox, the Greek Paradox, the East African paradox, the Swiss Paradox, the Pacific Island Paradox. These
countries have high levels of saturated fat consumption, but low
levels of heart disease. France has one of the highest—the French
consume four and a half times as much butter as US Americans,
for instance—but the French have substantially lower CHD.[60] The
Masai of Kenya eat a diet almost entirely of meat, milk, and blood.
On average, young Masai warriors ingest 300 grams of animal fat
every day. Yet their cholesterol levels are some of the lowest found
anywhere—averaging under 160—and heart disease is unknown.
On autopsy, atheromas (bad arterial plaques) were absent. George
Mann, the researcher who studied the Masai, was led by his findings
to declare the Lipid Hypothesis "the public health diversion of this
century ... the greatest scam in the history of medicine."[61]

A study of the Samburu tribe of Uganda yielded similar findings—neither heart disease nor elevated cholesterol levels, despite a
daily diet of 400g of animal fat. They also had no rheumatoid arthritis, degenerative arthritis, or high blood pressure.[62]

Another African pastoralist culture is the Kalenjins of Kenya.
Raw and fermented dairy products form the bulk of their diet. Not
only are they free of chronic and degenerative diseases, they are
world-renowned runners. "Athletes from this one tribe of 3 million
people have won 40 percent of all the highest international honors
available in men's distance running," in track, cross-country, and
road racing.[63] A Kalenjin has won the Boston Marathon four times
since 1988. Ron Schmid calls this "an indication of profound natural forces at work."[64]

Another epidemiological study discovered the Pacific Island
Paradox. Coconut is a staple food of the people of Pukapuka and
Tokelau, and coconut oil is more highly saturated than animal fats.
The two islands' inhabitants consumed 35% and 55%, respectively,

of their calories in the form of saturated fat. Cardiovascular disease was absent, as were degenerative diseases in general.[65] To quote Dr. Malcolm Kendrick, "I would just ask, how many paradoxes do you need before the only paradox left is the diet-heart hypothesis itself?"[66]

The Japanese? They've increased their consumption both of total fat and animal fat over 250 percent since 1961—and they are now *the longest living people in the world.* Stroke was the number one cause of death in the 1960s, but both stroke incidence and mortality from strokes declined rapidly from 1960 to 1975. And was there a dietary change during this period? Yes. Consumption of both animal protein and fat *increased* significantly, as one would expect during a time of economic prosperity. Blood cholesterol also increased, while blood pressure and strokes went down. To get even more specific, Japanese researchers tracked 3,700 people from 1984 to 2001, and those who ate the most animal fat had a "sixty-two percent lower risk of ischemic stroke death."[67]

Want more? A survey of 40,000 Japanese subjects found that over a sixteen-year period, "those who ate the most eggs, dairy products, and fish had a twenty-eight percent lower risk of stroke than those who ate the least."[68]

Then there's India, where the incidence of CHD was examined in over a million men. The highest CHD rates were in Madras, which is in southern India. The lowest rates were in Punjab, which is in the north. Their dietary difference? In disease-prone Madras, fat consumption was lower and consisted of polyunsaturated vegetable oils. In healthier Punjab, milk products supplied the fat, with only 2 percent coming from polyunsaturates. The Punjab men with their protective saturated fats were "seven times less likely to die from heart disease than those in Madras," and their overall life span was eight years longer. This, despite the fact that they smoked more.[69]

And then there's China. There is a bizarre and entrenched myth among the health-conscious in the West that the Chinese don't have cardiovascular disease. The idea is that they eat a lot of rice and vegetables and very little protein or fat, are healthy, and thus are living proof of the vegetarian myth. Write the Drs. Eades:

> However, the truth of the matter is that the Chinese do
> indeed have cardiovascular disease, and lots of it.... The rates
> of death from cardiovascular disease suffered by both rural
> and urban Chinese males is almost indistinguishable from
> the rate experienced by American males, while the rates
> of cardiovascular deaths for both rural and urban Chinese
> women is significantly higher than those suffered by American
> females.... The notion that the Chinese don't have disease of
> the heart and blood vessels is what we like to call a vampire
> myth—it simply refuses to die. The myth that low-fat, high-
> carbohydrate diets are healthy lives on and on.[70]

The difference between Chinese cardiovascular disease and cardiovascular disease in the US is simply the form it takes. In China, it's stroke; in the US, heart attack. For urban Chinese men, the rate of heart attack is about half that of US American men, but their rate of stroke is almost *six times higher*. For urban Chinese women, the heart attack rate is almost three-quarters the rate of US Americans and their stroke rate is about *five times higher*.[71]

Had enough? Who knows what other factors are involved with countries on the other side of the world, you might be saying defensively. Fine, let's look at the United States.

The past fifteen years have seen a reduction in fat consumption of almost 25 percent,[72] due to the relentless badgering of the medical establishment and the willingness of corporate food manufacturers to fabricate an endless array of faux-foods with their faux-fats: cheap polyunsaturated vegetable oils that have to be chemically altered to approach the mouthfeel that humans, craving our native saturated fats, will accept.

Twenty-five percent is a big reduction. Did you get healthier? Or did you notice that the incidence of diseases commonly blamed on animal products has gone from high to epidemic?

> Type 2 diabetes has increased by a factor of more than *ten*.
> Heart disease deaths, after more than ten years of decline,
> took a turn for the worse in 1992 and have slowly been in-

creasing since. An accurate measure of the increase in cardiovascular diseases can be seen in the rates of discharge from the
hospital of patients with that diagnosis, which, according to
the American Heart Association, have increased by 25 percent
since 1976. The incidence of stroke is on the rise, and cancer
continues its relentless and increasing toll with the very cancers most often blamed on fat consumption—cancer of the
breast and prostate—leading the charge.[73]

Some of the experts have noticed, and even publicly admitted,
that the dietary experiment inflicted on the US public has been an
utter failure.[74] William Willett of the Harvard School of Public
Health has said, "Low-fat has been like a religion. But it was just
a hypothesis to begin with."[75] We've done what they told us—ate
less fat, more carbohydrate—and have gotten sicker.

Or look at the famous Framingham Heart study. Started in
1948 to monitor the health of five thousand residents of a Boston
suburb, it attempted to examine the Lipid Hypothesis by measuring serum cholesterol levels and CHD. It's well worth reading the
whole study as an object lesson in denial. For example, *declining*
cholesterol levels in people over 50 were associated with *increases*
both in overall mortality and in death from CHD. "For every
1mg/dl per year drop in cholesterol levels during the first 14 years
of the Framingham study, there was a 14% increase in cardiovascular death and 11% increase in overall mortality during the
subsequent 18 years."[76] Yet the study is claimed by proponents of
the Lipid Hypothesis to prove the link between high cholesterol
and CHD.

And the role of saturated fat in Framingham? Dr. William
Castelli, the study's director, has written publicly that "In Framingham, Mass., the more saturated fat one ate, the more cholesterol one ate, the more calories one ate, the lower the person's serum
cholesterol ... We found that the people who ate the most cholesterol, ate the most saturated fat, ate the most calories, weighed the
least, and were the most physically active."[77]

Never mind the epidemiological studies. We don't like them anyway. What we really need is a rigorous, controlled study. Anthony Colpo describes what that perfect clinical trial would look like:

> Such a trial would compare a group of subjects of similar sex, age and health status, who have been randomly assigned to eat diets that are identical in every respect, except that one contains a significant amount of saturated fat (the control group), while the other contains a greatly reduced amount (the treatment group). Ideally, this trial would be 'double-blind', meaning that both researchers and participants would be unaware of who is in the treatment group and who is in the control group, a safeguard that would help prevent researcher bias and the possibility of a placebo effect amongst the subjects.[78]

In fact, such studies have been done, and done relentlessly, trying to prove some link between saturated fat, cholesterol, and CHD. Some of them meet standards that are scientifically rigorous; others must be read with a cautious and educated eye. The very first was designed by Lester M. Morrison in 1946. It specifically sought to investigate the relationship between the reduction of fat consumption and cardiac deaths. One hundred heart attack survivors were divided into two groups. The intervention group was placed on a calorie-restricted, low-fat, high-protein diet supplemented with calcium, phosphorus, brewer's yeast and wheat germ. At year eight, twenty-two of the intervention group had died while thirty-eight of the control subjects died.

Hopefully you can start to see the problem with this study. This was a multifaceted intervention, and there is no way to know which of the variables was the one that did the cardiac trick. The higher protein? That's been linked to lower CHD. Some members of the intervention group lost weight and that alone can improve cardiovascular profiles. We know that B vitamins—present in both the brewer's yeast and the wheat germ—lower levels of homocysteine, which is an atherogenic agent. Selenium is an antioxidant that may have clinical benefit for CHD patients, and yeast is a good source. Any of these variables could be responsible, and there's no way of knowing which one until each element is controlled. So when advocates of the Lipid Hypothesis hold up this particular study as evidence—and some of them do—feel free to know better.

The first clinical study on the Lipid Hypothesis that was blinded, randomized, and controlled—the first one, in other words, worth mentioning—was done in London, England, in 1965. Researchers took eighty volunteers and substituted corn oil for the saturated fat in their food. Notice: the fat was the only thing that changed. And the results? The corn oil people saw an average drop in serum cholesterol of 23 mg/dl. They also died. There were more "CHD incidents, deaths and total deaths" in the intervention group than in the control group. Another group was put on olive oil with results almost as bad. In the doctor's words, "under the circumstances of this trial corn oil cannot be recommended in the treatment of ischaemic heart disease. It is most unlikely to be beneficial, and it is possibly harmful."[79] Would that anyone had listened.

The first trial of the Lipid Hypothesis in the US was called the Anti-Coronary Club. Published in 1966, it compared eleven hundred men eating the "Prudent Diet" with a control group eating regularly. The Prudent Diet replaced saturated fat with polyunsaturated fat. The subjects' cholesterol levels dropped from an initial reading of 260 to an average of 225. These are the details the summary crows about. You might think the study had a happy ending—unless you kept reading. Nine months later, a second article revealed that eight of the prudent subjects died from heart attacks, while *none* of the control group did. Further, the total deaths on the Prudent Diet numbered twenty-six; only six men in the control group died. The deaths are basically ignored in the authors' discussion.[80] Which proves something beyond the fallacy of the Lipid Hypothesis, something about the inhuman rationality of science and the egos involved therein that many of us would rather not know.

Maybe you don't need to read all the studies, or all the books that debunk them. Maybe knowing that there are cultures consuming 80 percent of their calories in the form of saturated fat with no CHD is enough. Maybe in the bottom of your mind is the place where love is food and food is love and you can still see the color of your grandmother's kitchen. You always knew she was right: butter was good, margarine a disgrace. You had real food once, made for you by a woman who knew what children needed because *her* mother knew, the generations a Russian nesting doll of nourishing wisdom. Somebody fed you once. Let yourself remember: it was good.

Or maybe it's not that easy, surrounded as we are by voices of authority bearing down on us with yet another reminder that our appetites are dangerous, our bodily hungers a war we need to fight. That war, of course, will be endless, the profits to the corporate food oligarchs immense. There will never be room in their annual reports for the local and sustainable, the truly nourishing, just as there is no room for the inconvenient dead in their scientific summaries.

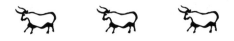

Know Your Fats, exhorts the title of Dr. Mary Enig's book on the subject. I wish it made a better bumper sticker. We need one. We need a countervailing resistance, an aggressive defense against all the forces lined up against our bodies and, in the end, our planet. Those forces turn out to be roughly the same. That knowledge was the crack in my vegan worldview that opened to the primary contradictions beneath. I couldn't grow the foods I was eating—lentils, rice, peanuts. Where did they come from? Didn't the people who grew those things need them? What right did I have to eat them? I soothed myself with a ritual obeisance to the amount of grain that animal foods required. I knew the global North had an economic stranglehold on the South, and that starvation was a painful way to die. As was being skinned alive at a slaughterhouse. Beyond that, all I knew was the choice between vegan and something worse: torture, murder. By the time I was twenty, I had grasped that agriculture with its annual grains was the end of the world. But the other choice was ... what? I wanted us all to be fed. I wanted women to be free and I wanted animals liberated. I wanted a world that was green and lush with the tendrilling of species. The vegans say they can get us there, that animal foods are a gluttony killing us and the planet. With no other visible options, I cast my lot with them.

And I was hungry. All the time. You can get plenty of calories and be deeply malnourished. To stay vegan, I had to fight a war with my hunger, a fact I would never have admitted, certainly not to myself, while I was doing it. If I had faced that animal craving full on, would I have had to stop being a vegan? Would my feminism, demanding as it must a cherishing loyalty to the female body as a baseline, have overruled it—especially since hunger is one of the main punishments that patriarchy inflicts on women for the crime of being female? I was a resistor of female abasement, not a participant, or at least not a willing one.

Instead I ignored the hunger, then denied it. And it didn't happen overnight: the deficits, the weary insulin receptors, the slow loss of vitality, the pain. The blood sugar crashes got worse with each year, until by the end I had to eat semi-constantly to feel like I wasn't about to die. All carbohydrate, of course, since that was all I allowed myself, which only guaranteed another crash. Meat was so taboo that craving protein would have been a hate crime akin to genocide. But my worst craving was for fat. For real fat. Not the vegetable oils I fried my tofu in, but the real thing: saturated fat.

Two years into being a vegan—two years in which not one molecule of animal fat passed into me—my mother put a bowl of dip on the table. This dip has been christened the Dairy Orgy Dip: it's sour cream and cream cheese with a few alliums for flavor.

I stared at that bowl. I couldn't stop staring at it. And I realized that nothing was going to stop me from eating it. Nothing I could remind myself, no fact, no image, was going to outweigh that biological urge. I ate. I remember thinking nothing: literally, no thoughts. Just hunger and its satiation.

Well-being flushed through me for the next few hours, starting somewhere in my brain. Not my mind, which was exhausted by the horror of what I'd done, but my actual brain. Twenty years later I would read the following and recognize myself. Captives from a prisoner of war camp were liberated and given a celebratory feast:

> The buffet was laden with roasts, vegetables, assorted breads, pies, salads, enticing deserts and fresh fruits, the likes of which they had not seen for several years. What did these men grab first? The butters, margarines, salad oils and creams. They were after fats. They consumed nothing else until the bare fats were gone.[81]

Clearly, I haven't had life experiences that even approach the level of trauma and deprivation in a war camp, and it would be insulting to those survivors to pretend otherwise. But the physical compulsion for fat, "the primordial craving for the substance,"[82] yes, I recognize that. You put your head down and you don't come up for air until the food—the fat—is gone. In that moment it's *better* than air. It's everything you could want, and the relief radiating from each mouthful tells you it's true: there's nothing better, nothing else, but this.

My vegan time is punctuated by those moments. "Binges" we called them, or "lapses," thus identifying them as a moral weakness, a political slippage, not a starved body, a shriveled brain, overriding a mind's ideological demands.

There was a small cafe that I used to pass every morning. They sold bagels cheap. I bought one. The next morning I knew what I was going to do without letting myself know: I got one with cream cheese. And the next day? I'll let you guess. I tried to pretend it wasn't happening, made myself throw away the memory with the tissue paper wrapping. Then I got one with double cream cheese. *Oh, god,* something in my brain woke and moaned. I couldn't stop. I also couldn't admit full on what I was doing, because then I'd *have* to stop. Guilt flooded my mind like relief flooded my body. What was wrong with me? Was I forgetting everything I knew, becoming one of them, a sell-out, a callous participant in torture? The veal crates, the cows chained to stalls, the willful cruelty of men: it was all there, inside that bagel. And I kept buying them, on and off, for about two months. I couldn't fathom what was happening to me, and like many vegans I've known, I tried to identify the cause as emotional. To admit it was a simple, physical need for a necessary nutrient would destroy our world and our identities. Therefore, these cravings, these lapses, had to be either emotional or spiritual, though that last wasn't a word we used. Still, that's the cultural framework handed down from Christianity. Bless me, sisters, for I have sinned: mea culpa, mea vegan culpa. I was falling away from God, a different god to be sure, but one I loved.

In the end I switched my route to remove the temptation, having learned nothing.

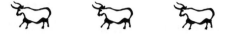

Here is the chemistry of fat. Fatty acids are carbon atoms linked together, with hydrogen atoms filling in where they can. A fat is called saturated when each of the potential carbon bonds is filled with a hydrogen atom. Their atoms form a straight line and fit together nicely; that's why they're solid at room temperature. Saturation makes them stable, which means they don't go rancid even when heated. Our bodies can make saturated fat from carbohydrates.

Monounsaturated fats are missing two hydrogen atoms. This gives their form a bend, so they don't pack together as tightly as the saturated fats. Think of olive or peanut oil: at room temperature they're liquid, but refrigerated they firm up. The human body can make monounsaturates from saturated fats.

Polyunsaturated fats are missing four or more hydrogens. They've got enough kinks in their form that they don't fit together well. Hence they're always liquid, and they are unstable. That means they go rancid very quickly and should never be heated. These are the vegetable oils—corn, soy—that began flooding our food supply in the 1920s.

Polyunsaturates in our food come mostly in two forms: omega-6 and omega-3. Since we can't make these they are "essential."

All dietary fats contain varying proportions of saturates, monounsaturates, and polyunsaturates. Coconut and palm oil contain the most saturated fat, with coconut at 92 percent. In contrast, butter is about 60 percent saturated fat, beef is 50 percent and lard about 40 percent.[83]

Fats are also classified by length. Short-chain fatty acids are only four to six carbon atoms long. On the other end of the spectrum are the very-long-chain fatty acids, which have twenty to twenty-four carbon atoms. Your body uses them to make prostaglandins, and some are also crucial to the health of the nervous system. Most important, some of us can synthesize very-long-chain fatty acids from other EFAs (essential fatty acids), but some of us can't. These people don't produce the enzymes for the task. They're called "obligate carnivores" and they must get their elongated fatty acids from animal products. If you come from a long line of island or coastal people who ate fish, this may well be you.

Vitamins A, D, E, and K are all called fat-soluble. They can only be transported by fat, and their absorption is partial at best without the presence of dietary fat. Further, these vitamins are only available in dietary fat. True vitamin A, writes lipid expert Mary Enig, "occurs only in foods of animal origin and requires fat for absorption."[84]

There are no plant sources of vitamin A. Plants contain proto-vitamin A, which must be converted to vitamin A. Even healthy adults can't do this efficiently, and the young and the old may not be able to do it at all. And without, in Enig's words, "adequate animal fats," none of us can.[85] Vitamin A is needed for "successful reproduction, normal cell division, vision ... functioning of the immune system, bone remodeling, the formation of enamel on teeth during their development in childhood, and skin health."[86]

Vitamin D regulates calcium absorption. And vitamin D begins life as ... cholesterol. Yes, the Evil One. You read that right. Cholesterol goes through a series of transformations, starting with sunlight on the skin. It is possible to get vitamin D from ingested sources alone, which is how humans survive in the arctic. All food sources of vitamin D are animal products: cod liver oil, other animal livers, egg yolks, fatty fish, and butter. Women living under the Taliban, who could only leave the house if covered from head to foot in a burkha, literally died from lack of vitamin D. In the West, vitamin D deficiencies are now widespread due to avoidance of direct sunlight and use of sunscreens. And truly dangerous deficiencies are seen in these three groups: very dark-skinned people living in far northern climates; girl children whose parents entomb them in cloth for cultural reasons; and vegans, especially their children.[87] Rickets is the disease caused by vitamin D deficiency; its main symptom is soft, deformed bones of the legs. Please listen: in one study, 28 percent of vegan children had rickets in the summer, and in winter, it was 55 percent.[88]

Vitamin E is necessary for reproduction and for cardiovascular health. It's also an important antioxidant. There are both plant and animal sources of vitamin E. Vitamin K is essential for blood clotting, and for supporting good bone density. Food sources include liver as well as leafy vegetables.

Vitamins A, D, B, and K are all essential to human health, and they need saturated fat for transportation and absorption. Vitamin A and D are especially linked to saturated fat since they're only available in animal foods.

We also need saturated fat to provide cholesterol. Some people claim that cholesterol isn't essential because our bodies can synthesize it. But the reason we can produce it is because we need so much of it. Explains Dr. Enig, "It is not possible for humans to eat enough cholesterol-containing foods every day to supply the amount that a human needs." [89] She continues, "The statement 'even if you didn't eat any cholesterol, your liver would manufacture enough for your body's needs' has been made so frequently it is often believed. But in fact, there is evidence that for some people cholesterol is an absolute dietary essential because their own synthesis is not adequate."[90]

Infants especially need cholesterol and saturated fat for their developing brains and nervous systems. Human breast milk is a rich source of cholesterol, as are cow's milk and goat's milk. Soy milk contains none. You may have noticed the little label on your soy milk that says "Not for use as an infant formula." That label is there because a set of naive parents, encouraged by their idiot midwife, exclusively fed their baby soy milk until she was severely malnourished, while another baby girl fed soy milk was admitted to the hospital with "heart failure, rickets, vasculitis and neurological damage."[91]

Our organs are surrounded by saturated fat both for protection and for fuel. This is especially true of our hearts. Under stress, the heart can draw on the highly saturated fat that encases it. In fact, fat is the preferred fuel of our hearts.

Dr. Kendrick took the data collected by the World Health Organization regarding saturated-fat consumption and heart-disease in Europe and created his own "14 Country Study" (see Figure 4E). He compared the seven countries with the lowest consumption of saturated fat to the seven countries with the highest consumption of saturated fat. The data are unequivocal: "Every single one of the seven countries with the lowest saturated-fat consumption has significantly higher rates of heart disease than every single one of the seven countries with the highest saturated-fat consumption.... [T]here is no connection between saturated fat consumption and heart disease."[92]

You don't want to trust these broad spectrum population studies? Fine. But at some point you have to admit: we have been lied to. Meanwhile, for five years running, Lipitor has been the best-selling pharmaceutical in the world.[93]

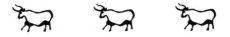

Fat is also preferred by our nervous systems. Without fat, our neurotransmitters literally can't transmit. Twenty-five percent of the body's cholesterol is in the brain, the brain that is made up of over 60 percent saturated fat. The brain's glial cells play a primary role in cognitive function: they provide "a substance that allows ... synapses to form, and function. Without this substance your brain would be almost entirely useless."[94] The name of this wonder substance? Cholesterol.

Low cholesterol also means low serotonin levels, which mean depression. Cholesterol is essential for the brain's serotonin receptors.[95] In fact, people on low-fat diets are *twice* as likely to die from suicide or violent death.[96] Dr. Beatrice Golomb did a detailed review of all the studies published since 1965 that examined a potential link between low cholesterol levels and violence. In her opinion, the correlation is causal.[97]

Clinical studies in rigorously controlled environments have also found that low-fat diets increase anger, depression, and anxiety.[98] Low cholesterol levels occur "more often amongst criminals, individuals diagnosed with violent or aggressive conduct disorders, homicidal offenders with histories of violence and suicide attempts related to alcohol, and people with poorly internalized social norms and low self-control."[99]

Here's an example of a well-controlled study. British researchers did an experiment on "a psychologically robust group who had never previously suffered from depression or anxiety, and who were not going through any 'stressful' events during the study." One group ate 41 percent fat; the other 25 percent fat. All meals were supplied to the volunteers by the researchers. In the interest of double-blinding, the foods were chosen to be as similar as possible. Then they switched, so that the low-fat dieters ate the high-fat diets, and vice versa. Each volunteer went through thorough psychological testing before and after each dietary trial.

The results?

> [W]hile ratings of anger-hostility slightly declined during the high-fat diet period, they significantly increased during the low-fat, high-carbohydrate diet period! Similarly, ratings of depression declined slightly during the high-fat period, but increased during the low-fat period ... Levels of attention-anxiety declined during the high-fat period, but did not change during the four weeks of low-fat eating.[100]

There are two things going on here. One is that the human body and its brain need saturated fat and cholesterol. The other is that while polyunsaturated fatty acids (PUFAs) are essential (the body can't make them) they are only needed in tiny amounts. The quantities currently consumed in the US damage both body and brain. Somewhere around 4 percent of our total calories should be polyunsaturates, with maybe 1.5 percent omega-3s and 2.5 percent omega-6s. Some experts suggest that the best ratio of Omega-3s to Omega-6s would be one to one.[101] These are the amounts found naturally in foods from nuts to greens to animal fat. Until very recently in human history, *no one* used discrete polyunsaturated vegetable oils, or at least not for food. They were used to make glue and paint. But corporate America took control of the food stream and flooded it with cheap, industrially produced oils and carbohydrates. And we've been drowning in degenerative diseases ever since. Those eating the standard US American diet—with its fitting acronym of SAD—get 30 percent of their calories from PUFAs. This is an experiment that's never been done before, and we are its subjects.

High consumption of PUFAs "has been shown to contribute to a large number of disease conditions including increased cancer and heart disease, immune system dysfunction, damage to the liver, reproductive organs, and lungs, digestive disorders, depressed learning ability, impaired growth, and weight gain."[102] A big problem with PUFAs is their tendency to oxidize, i.e., go rancid, when exposed to air, moisture, or heat—like, say, when they're used for cooking. Whereas saturated oils are stable because every carbon is paired with a hydrogen, the PUFAs are exactly the opposite. They've got free radicals everywhere. Technically speaking, they have "single atoms or clusters with an unpaired electron in an outer orbit."[103] The take-away point is they're looking for a fight. They attack cell membranes and blood cells, destroying DNA sequences. That spells cancer when it happens in organs. When it happens in the blood vessels, it causes damage that must be repaired before you spring a leak, especially as blood vessels are under pressure. And that is how plaquing begins: with damage to the arteries that cholesterol—the body's repair substance—tries to patch. Cholesterol doesn't just gum up your arteries for no reason. It's there because something's wrong. "Cholesterol," explain Sally Fallon and Mary Enig, is "manufactured in large amounts when the arteries are irritated or weak." To use their apt metaphor, blaming cholesterol for CHD is like blaming the fire fighters for the fire.[104]

Whether the damage is caused by sugar and insulin, as discussed previously, or by PUFAs and their free radicals, it's cholesterol that *keeps* us from dying—and then takes the blame for killing us. Just in case you need more convincing, only 26 percent of the fat in arterial plaques is saturated. The balance is unsaturated, and the majority of that is polyunsaturated.[105]

The PUFAs have been indicted in autoimmune and inflammatory diseases, among them arthritis, Parkinson's, and Alzheimer's. Part of the underlying problem is that commercial vegetable oils contain large amounts of omega-6 fatty acids and almost no omega-3s. The omega-6s create "inflammation, high blood pressure, irritation of the digestive tract, depressed immune function, sterility, cell proliferation ... [and] cancer."[106] As if that wasn't enough, they interfere with the synthesis of prostaglandins.

Prostawhat? Technically, prostaglandins are hormones. They are found in almost all animal tissues and organs and they have a huge array of effects. For instance, prostaglandins

- cause constriction or dilatation in vascular smooth muscle cells
- cause aggregation or disaggregation of platelets
- sensitize spinal neurons to pain
- regulate inflammatory mediation
- regulate calcium movement
- control hormone regulation
- control cell growth.[107]

And they're synthesized from fatty acids—from dietary fat. That fact should make it obvious why eating the wrong fats would result in disrupted prostaglandins.

Meanwhile insufficient omega-3s can cause "cancer, depression ... diabetes, arthritis, allergies, asthma and dementia."[108] Omega-3 deficiencies are also implicated in high blood pressure, heart attack, and stroke. Omega-3s are almost entirely absent from the US American diet. According to Jo Robinson, "twenty percent of Americans have levels so low that they defy detection."[109] The best sources should be eggs, fish, meat, and dairy, but they no longer are. Why? Because factory farming stuffs animals full of grain, which changes the composition of their body fat. Yes, grain again. Grain is desperately low in omega-3s and high in omega-6s. Hens on pasture eating insects, small mammals, and green plants will produce eggs with a stellar omega-6 to omega-3 ratio: one to one. In sad contrast, the eggs from confined hens fed grain can have *nineteen times* more omega-6 than omega-3.[110] Grass is a rich source of omega-3s, so rich that products from a pasture-fed cow can have an omega-6 to -3 ratio ranging from three to one to less than one to one. Compare that to her grain-stuffed sister whose ratio may be as high as *fourteen to one*.[111]

This is what agriculture, especially agriculture condensed to corporate America and the grain cartels, has done to us.

Currently, 40 percent of all our dead are killed by CHD. Yet at the same time that the proportion of animal fats in the fats consumed by people in the US dropped from 83 percent to 62 percent, the consumption of vegetable oils exploded *400 percent*.[112] Julia Ross, in her crucial book *The Mood Cure*, points out that polyunsaturated vegetable oils

> have even crept into important foods that used to be almost totally omega-6 free. Fish, meats, and poultry are now raised on high-omega-6 grains instead of low-omega-3 algae, grass, and bugs. There is no question that ever increasing rates of depression, heart disease, and cancer have been the direct results. The Japanese and Israeli scientific communities have concluded, after several decades of consuming these "Western" oils and suffering epidemic increases in "Western" diseases as a consequence, that the high-omega-6 vegetable oils have been a disaster for their people. A grim report to the National Institutes of Health by the top Japanese experts concluded that omega-6 vegetable oils "are inappropriate for human use as foods."[113]

You tell me what to blame: the saturated fats we've always eaten—for four million years—or the industrially manufactured oils that until recently were used in paint.

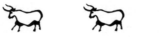

Dr. Weston Price was a dentist who practiced in Cleveland, Ohio. He was born on a farm in Ontario, Canada, and received his degree in 1893. This date is important, as he entered the field just prior to the glut of industrial food. Over the course of the next thirty years, he watched children's dentition—and indeed their overall health—deteriorate. There were suddenly children whose teeth didn't fit inside their mouths, children with foreshortened jaws, children with lots of cavities. Not only were their dental arches too small, but he noticed their nasal passages were also too narrow, and they had poor health overall: asthma, allergies, behavioral problems. His hypothesis was that these deformities and deteriorations were caused by nutritional deficits. To test his hypothesis, he and his wife, Florence, a nurse, traveled the globe looking for cultures that achieved perfect health in their members. In the 1930s, such cultures still existed. He also found people whose kin had abandoned their traditional foods for "the displacing foods of our modern civilization" with the same results everywhere.[114] Namely, cavities and shrunken dental arches, skeletal deformities, cancer, and the full complement of degenerative diseases. Price took meticulous notes on people's diets. He also took samples of their foods for analysis. And maybe most importantly, he took pictures. In his report on his travels, *Nutrition and Physical Degeneration*, he wrote:

> In presenting the evidence I am utilizing photographs very liberally. A good illustration is said to be equivalent to a thousand words of text.... The pictures are much more convincing than words can be, and since the text challenges many of the current theories, the most conclusive evidence available is essential.[115]

It was essential for me. Having once read the text, I didn't return to it. It was the photos I went back to, over and over. The perfect string-of-pearls teeth in the parents leaned and twisted in their children. It was like an earthquake had run through their jaws. Well, it had, but not just through their jaws—through their whole culture. And their degenerating health was one of the horrible results.

Price found a number of remote groups for study. He was looking for perfect health: freedom from dental decay and from chronic, degenerative, and infectious diseases across generations. He examined the teeth and overall health of Swiss people in the Alps and Gaels on the Outer Hebrides, Inuit and Cree peoples in North America, and Melanesians and Polynesians in the South Pacific. The Prices traveled over 6,000 miles in Africa and studied thirty tribes. Of those thirty, six evinced the sturdy health he was seeking.

Price found a range of human cultures from hunter-gatherers to pastoralists to agriculturalists, and a wide variety of foodstuffs. Dr. Ron Schmid, author of *Native Nutrition: Eating According to Ancestral Wisdom*, writes:

> Tribes eating grains-based natural-foods diets had well-formed dental arches and resistance to infectious diseases, but their physical development, resistance to dental decay, and strength were inferior to tribes eating more animal-source foods. The people strongest physically and often 100 percent resistant to dental diseases were herdsmen-hunter-fisherman. In towns and ports where some groups ate a combination of refined and primitive foods, problems developed, but not to the extent occurring when native foods were abandoned entirely.[116]

Price saw the same pattern in Australia, where coastal Aborigines eating seafood were the healthiest. When their diet was displaced by refined agricultural food, "tuberculosis and crippling arthritis became common."[117]

The Prices also found perfect health in Torres Strait islanders. The government physician for the islanders stated that in his thirteen years among the native population of four thousand, he had never seen cancer. He had operated on several dozen malignancies among the white population of about three hundred. In fact, among the indigenous, any conditions requiring surgery were extremely rare.[118] The indigenous people resisted assimilation, especially to industrial food. They understood that government stores were a danger, and on a number of occasions almost took up violence against such stores.[119] Would that the rest of us would follow their lead.

In New Zealand, the Prices met with Maori people at all stages of assimilation to Westernization and documented the same decay of health and increasing vulnerability to chronic and degenerative diseases.

The brilliance of Dr. Price was that he was able to recognize the pattern. He wasn't distracted by the variations in macronutrients or by differences in basic foodstuffs. He was able to identify the dietary principles that granted perfect immunity to chronic and degenerative diseases. Writes Schmid, "Price gave us overwhelming evidence of natural laws concerning dietary needs, laws that operate in human beings everywhere to regulate immunity, reproduction and virtually every other aspect of health."[120]

What "immune" people universally valued were nutrient-dense animal fats: organ meats, bone marrow, fish oils and roe, egg yolks, lard, butter. Liver was especially valued, often eaten raw, and sometimes considered sacred. Schmid writes that "foods from one or more of six different groups were absolutely essential." The essential groups were:

1. Seafood: fish and shellfish, fish organs, fish liver oils and fish eggs.
2. Organ meats from wild animals or grass-fed domestic animals.
3. Insects.
4. Fats of certain birds and monogastric (one-stomach) animals such as sea mammals, Guinea pigs, bears and hogs.
5. Egg yolks from pastured chickens and other birds.
6. Whole milk, cheese and butter from grass-fed animals.[121]

When Price analyzed these foods—he collected over 10,000 samples—he discovered that the immune groups were eating *over ten times* more vitamin A and vitamin D than the US Americans of his time. These vitamins are found exclusively in animal fats. Their food also provided over four times more minerals and water soluble vitamins. Writes author and activist Sally Fallon, "Price referred to the fat-soluble vitamins as 'catalysts' or 'activators' upon which the assimilation of all the other nutrients depended—protein, minerals and vitamins. In other words, without the dietary factors found in animal fats, all the other nutrients largely go to waste."[122]

Price has been proven right, if anybody is listening. Vitamins A, D, K, and E are only available in animal fats, and those fats are necessary for minerals to be absorbed and for protein to be digested.

Other doctors have also observed the near-universal perfect health of hunter-gatherers. Dr. Edward Howell, a pioneer in enzyme research, reported on another doctor who lived with the indigenous people near Aklavik (northern Canada), stating, "He has never seen a single case of malignancy."[123] One report from a doctor who examined hundreds of indigenous people on their native diets found that "there were no signs of any heart disease ... No case of cancer or diabetes."[124] Such observations are common in the anthropological literature and are completely ignored by the medical institutions that control the public health policies of our country.

In 1933, Price interviewed Dr. Josef Romig, a surgeon who served both the traditional and assimilated native people in Alaska for thirty-six years. "Cancer was unknown" among the traditional indigenous—he had "never seen a case." When they took up the foods of the civilized—flour, sugar, vegetable oil—"it frequently occurred."[125] When assimilated people contracted tuberculosis, Romig prescribed returning to their "native conditions and the native nutrient-dense diet."[126] Tuberculosis was usually fatal on civilized foods, but often cured on their indigenous diet. That diet consisted of "whale, caribou, musk ox, Arctic hare, rock ptarmigan, walrus, seal, polar bear, seagulls, geese, duck, auks, and fish, all often (but not always) eaten raw and fermented."[127] They also ate liberally of salmon and roe. Organ meats of large land mammals were also consumed raw. Plant foods eaten were mostly sorrel grasses and flower blossoms preserved in seal oil and the fermented stomach contents of caribou.

The raw components of these fats are critical. The metabolism of cooked fats results in by-products called ketone bodies. An elevated number of ketone bodies in the blood and urine is a state called ketosis. The levels of ketone bodies in people eating low-carb diets like the Atkins diet are an endless source of controversy. If the low-carb detractors in both the medical profession and the media knew their biology a little bit better, they'd drop it. Journalist Gary Taubes interviewed ketosis experts for his groundbreaking *New York Times* article, "What If It's All Been a Big Fat Lie?" The experts "universally sided with Atkins, and suggested that maybe the medical community and the media confuse ketosis with ketoacidosis, a variant of ketosis that occurs in untreated diabetics and can be fatal." Ketosis is a perfectly natural state. We evolved to store fat when we had plenty, and burn fat when food was slim. "Rather than being poison, which is how the press often refers to ketones, they make the body run more efficiently and provide a backup fuel source for the brain," explains Taubes. One expert "has shown that both the heart and brain run 25 percent more efficiently on ketones than on blood sugar."[128] Which should make you wonder if they aren't in the end the fuel we were designed for.

But what is more interesting is that studies of indigenous people eating essentially nothing but protein and fat "showed no ketosis. These native people completely metabolized the fats in their high-protein and high-fat diet because many of the fats were raw. This is not surprising since lipase [an enzyme for fat digestion] is found in concentrated amounts in raw, natural fats."[129] Humans have only been eating cooked foods for some 200,000 years, a blink of an evolutionary eye. Those members of our species who remembered the value of raw fats—with their enzymes, their intact vitamins—are the ones who have kept the human template undiminished. When Price asked immune groups why they ate the foods they did, the reply was always the same: "So we can make perfect babies."[130]

There were finer points to Price's discoveries. Immune groups ate some fermented foods, which are full of enzymes and pro-biotics; especially nutritious foods were eaten by prospective parents; and any seeds (nuts, grains, tubers) that were eaten were soaked, sprouted, and/or fermented to disable the antinutrients. Phytates, for instance, are present in all seeds including nuts, legumes, and grains. They are one of the plant world's basic self-defense mechanisms. Remember that, generally speaking, plants don't want to be eaten either, but they use chemicals instead of locomotion. Phytates bind with minerals in the eater's digestive tract, making the minerals inaccessible. Minerals, especially calcium, are needed for digestion. The body loans itself calcium from accessible storage spots like teeth and bones, on the theory that the food ingested will pay it back. Eating is a promise we make our bodies, and it's a promise we break each time we eat processed foods, like white flour and sugar, that have had their minerals removed mechanically, or untreated seeds like the whole grains being pushed on us as "healthy" from every direction.

Seeds soaked in warm water are fooled into thinking that conditions are ripe for growth. They disable their phytates and their tiny radicles begin their tentative search for soil. People all around the world have figured out ways to make seeds more digestible through sprouting, rinsing and fermenting them. Traditional sourdough breads are one example. The long preparation process that some Native American tribes use on acorns is another.

There are also cultures that are missing that knowledge. The widespread use of flat breads made from whole, untreated wheat in the Middle East results in stunted growth and short adult stature: there are too many phytates removing too many minerals in their diets.

Of course the food with the most minerals are marine foods, which is why the healthiest people Price found were coastal-dwelling fishing peoples. First runner-up would be land-based mammals, which explains why the hunter-gatherers and pastoralists placed next.

And me? I came in last. Price looked specifically for indigenous groups that achieved perfect health on plant foods only. He found none. "It is significant," he wrote, "that I have as yet found no group that was building and maintaining good bodies exclusively on plant foods. A number of groups are endeavoring to do so with marked evidence of failure."[131]

And there I was, with my spine coming apart at the seams for no apparent reason, staring at his photographs. No one in those cultures had my disease. Perfect teeth, perfect bones. They had no arthritis, no degenerative conditions. Understand the pain level I was living in by then: I couldn't sit for more than thirty minutes or stand for more than ten. Every daily task had to be broken down into the smallest activities, separated by endless stretches of lying down. One extra load of laundry or a long line at the bank and pain would eat my life to the bone. I could spend weeks lying in bed, waiting for it to subside.

And here were these pictures. Fourteen cultures where teeth and bones held through their lives, all the way to the end. It was their food that carried them through. And I ate precisely the opposite. Information began to crystallize, like freeze-up on a lake. There was an exact moment when knowledge took hold, and it was cold clean through: I had done this to myself. And there was no way back.

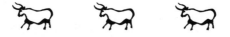

Take all the information I've laid out about fats, about how PUFAs hurt your brain and saturated fats help it, how omega-6s are implicated and omega-3s are missing. Now, combine that with the poor-quality plant protein of vegetarian and especially vegan diets. Your brain would like you to know that all of your neurotransmitters are made from amino acids. Whatever happiness you've been allotted in life will only be felt through protein.

Tryptophan, for instance, is the amino acid precursor for serotonin. And, as nutritionist Julia Ross points out, "Most vegetable foods contain much less tryptophan than animal-derived foods."[132]

Even vegans talk about "the vegan police." Admit you know what I'm talking about: aggressive, rigid, on a hair trigger, and in a semi-constant state of rage. That's what happens to a human with a brain deprived of protein and fat. I had a full-blown anxiety disorder by the time I was done, and I lost most of my youth to the dull, gray nothing of depression. Rage was all I had left to feel, and feel it I did, but it was exhausting. When the tiniest task is inexplicably overwhelming, and the world is all surface, repulsive and flat, the self is a cage. No amount of will can melt it, because it's a biological reality. Hence the fat binges, the cravings. It will only change when the brain is allowed to consume what it needs.

If you spend any time with vegans, you will notice their intense sugar cravings. One of my colleagues wrote,

> A bunch of my vegan friends would eat candy and make disgustingly sugary concoctions of various kinds. Things like cherry pasta in chocolate sauce. And then later I figured they probably craved sugar because of their various nutrient deficiencies.[133]

They're craving sugar for three reasons. The first is that on a diet of carbohydrate, they're bound to be hypoglycemic, and when blood sugar is falling, there is a terrible imperative to get it back up. And because their food doesn't contain any quality protein, their brains are desperate for serotonin and endorphins. Endorphins are a collection of brain chemicals that "transmit enjoyment, contentment, and euphoria ... They ... amplify pleasure and make pain tolerable."[134] Falling in love produces an endorphin high. So does chocolate, as it contains PEA (phenylethylamine), one of the aminos from which the brain builds endorphins. "Endorphin building," explains Julia Ross, "requires a big, consistent supply of high-protein foods like fish, eggs, cottage cheese, and chicken."[135]

Without those high-protein foods, your brain can't produce endorphins. But a sugar hit will trigger an adrenaline rush which sends your endorphin levels up temporarily.

And anyone who isn't eating enough good quality protein is also at risk for serotonin depletion—i.e., depression—from simple lack of tryptophan. Even the good sources of tryptophan have been virtually destroyed by industrial agriculture. There should be more tryptophan than there is in our meat, eggs, and dairy: probably three times as much. In CAFOs, animals are fed grains, especially corn, which is low in tryptophan. Hence, the animal products that should keep our brains happy are deficient once again because of grain and factory farming. Julia Ross points out that "tryptophan has been diminishing from our food supply for the past one hundred years, about as long as our rate of depression has been climbing."[136] And of course eating grains produces the same low-tryptophan state in us that it does in other animals.

What does this have to do with sugar? Eating sugar triggers a flood of insulin. Insulin moves through your bloodstream, sweeping up sugars, fats, and amino acids, and transporting them into your cells for storage. The only substance that insulin can't lock onto is tryptophan. With all the other amino acids out of the way, tryptophan suddenly has no competition in crossing the blood-brain barrier. Hence, for a brief time, a serotonin-deprived brain gets some desperately needed tryptophan. It's why depressed people crave sweets and starchy "comfort foods." And it's only during those short lacunas that a vegan's brain feels normal.

The third reason vegans crave sugar is to combat the exhaustion. We don't have a word in English that encapsulates the concept of vital force or life energy. In Hindi, it's called "prana." In Chinese medicine, it's called "chi." Whatever you call it, it's very real. So is the bone-aching exhaustion that comes when you use it up. And if you're not eating meat, you're using up your own stores. There's a tipping point for all of us: once that vital energy is gone, you don't get it back. One main reason vegetarians start eating meat is the exhaustion. "Some people say they actually felt worse on a vegetarian diet," reports an article in *Vegetarian Times*. Of course the author takes it as self-evident that this can't be true: such people simply "weren't eating balanced meals."[137]

I've read the vegan message boards on this subject. I've seen the vegans' contempt. The posters, of course, can't let themselves believe that a vegetarian diet might cause harm to anyone's body: we all can and should be vegetarian, if not vegan, and anyone who suggests otherwise is a heretic. "They just want to eat easy food at McDonald's," was one message. "They're looking for an excuse for their cowardice," wrote another.

I haven't eaten at McDonalds in almost thirty years. And I will live in life-altering pain for the rest of my days because I believed and believed and believed in veganism. No one could have been more dedicated. Six weeks into it I felt tired. Tired faded into exhaustion. Exhaustion turned to winter—always winter, never Christmas—at the marrow of me.[138] Yet I kept at it for twenty years.

So here's a deal. Try living in my body for ten minutes. Then you can call me a coward.

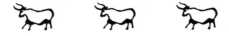

How did this happen? How did the traditional foods recognized as essential, if not sacred, since forever get demonized by our culture? That history has been documented by writers like Gary Taubes and Ron Schmid, and a full recounting is beyond the scope of this book.[139] But a brief overview should help the reader understand the brute financial interests involved, and what corporate profits have cost the rest of us.

Schmid titles his chapter on the subject "Betrayal." "Betrayal," he writes, "is a strong word, implying disloyalty, treachery, deliberately misleading behavior. My premise ... is that many of our private and public institutions have betrayed our trust."[140] That betrayal has happened for the same reason that it usually does: money. Agriculture and the food industry are a vast component of the US economy—$1 trillion in annual sales, which is 13 percent of the gross national product.[141] Explains Schmid:

> The growth of the food industry was coincident with a gradual but wholesale change in the typical American diet, from one based on locally grown whole foods to one based on processed foods that may come from anywhere. As the industry grew, farming as a lifestyle declined; forty percent of Americans lived on farms in 1900, compared to less than two percent today.... Fifty years ago, hundreds of thousands of farmers raised small flocks of chickens. Today, a few corporations produce nearly all our chickens through a system known as vertical integration: a single corporation owns all stages of

production and marketing.... Most people today don't realize
that chicken used to taste very different.[142]

Nor do we realize what's happened to our land, our communities, and our food. When Schmid says "locally grown food" that
means an actual farmer raised it, instead of a corporate-owned
factory producing it. That farmer would have been your neighbor,
a member of your faith community, an official on your local school
board. You knew each other; for better or for worse, you needed
each other. There was a moral economy of social capital that un-
derlay the economic exchanges. Those local communities and the
bonds of care they both created and depended on have been destroyed by the corporate takeover of our food supply. Look at the
numbers Schmid supplies: local farmers are down from 40 percent
to 2 percent. And those 2 percent, growing price-fixed commodities
and committing suicide, might as well be serfs.

Forcing the farmer off the farm has also meant taking the animals off it. The most efficient way to produce industrial food is on
huge plantations of monocrops, fertilized by fossil fuel, with the animals—now animal units—crammed into confinement operations
and crammed full of cheap corn. The environmental nightmare of
fertilizer run-off—dead zones in the ocean, bacterial contamination
of groundwater, and topsoil loss—has been one result. The moral
nightmare of factory farming should be obvious to anyone with a
pulse.

It's the economics of industrial food production that drive all
this destruction. Taubes explains that starches and refined carbohydrates are "calorie for calorie ... the cheapest nutrients for the food
industry to produce, and they can be sold at the highest profit."[143]
The corn in your cornflakes accounts for less than 10 percent of the
retail cost: sometimes the packaging costs more than the ingredients. Meanwhile, the production of animal foods like beef, chicken,
and eggs cost 50 to 60 percent of their retail price.[144] Isn't it obvious where the people in control of the food stream would like to
shift our diets? Those cheap carbohydrates have been the source of
enormous profits.

And that shift in the US diet was given a huge boost by government policy recommendations. The first boost came in 1977 from a Senate committee headed by George McGovern. The second came in 1984 when the National Institutes of Health endorsed a low-fat diet. In between, hundreds of millions of public dollars were spent on five huge studies that tried to link dietary fat and CHD. Those studies were abysmal failures.[145] And some scientists knew ahead of time that they would be. Phil Handler, the president of the National Academy of Scientists, asked Congress, "What right has the federal government to propose that the American people conduct a vast nutritional experiment, with themselves as subjects, on the strength of so very little evidence that it will do them any good?"[146] Dr. Pete Aherns, an expert on cholesterol metabolism, told the McGovern committee that the effects of a low-fat diet weren't a scientific matter but "a betting matter."[147]

It's twenty-five years later and we aren't winning this bet. Each US American now eats sixty pounds more grain per annum and thirty pounds more of cheap sugars, mostly from corn. One result is that adult-onset diabetes can't be called that anymore because so many kids have it. Our food supply has also been stripped of nourishing fats like butter, lard, and coconut oil, which have been replaced by the grain cartels' cheap, rancid vegetable oils, all with the stamp of healthy, low-fat approval. Note well that those "healthy," low-fat substances include hydrogenated oils, chemically altered fats for which there are in fact no safe levels of consumption.

Alan Stone, staff director for the McGovern committee, told Gary Taubes that

> he had an inkling about how the food industry would respond to the new dietary goals back when the hearings were first held. An economist pulled him aside, he said, and gave him a lesson on market disincentives to healthy eating: "He said if you create a new market with a brand-new manufactured food, give it a brand-new fancy name, put a big advertising budget behind it, you can have a market all to yourself and force your competitors to catch up. You can't do that with

fruits and vegetables. It's harder to differentiate an apple from an apple."[148]

The food industry has developed over 100,000 new processed foods since 1990. First, let's acknowledge that "developing new foods" is a bizarre and rather frightening concept—and eating them even more so. Next, understand the implications of the fact that fully a quarter of them are "nutritionally enhanced" products that can claim endorsements of health by virtue of being low-fat or cholesterol-free or higher in calcium.[149] Try to comprehend the scale of this: food companies spend $33 billion a year in advertising.[150] What they put their money on is the lowest cost, highest priced items—the unmitigated junk—that they can now market as "heart-healthy" since they're all sugar and no fat. Pepsico alone spends over a billion dollars a year pushing sugar and hydrogenated vegetable oils on the US American public, including children.

The food industry also spends money, lots and lots of money, to influence doctors, nutritionists, and the universities that train them. Professional meetings of such experts are "overtly sponsored" by industrial food giants, which also fund travel expenses and honoraria.[151] They also fund the professional journals: the *Journal of the American Society of Clinical Nutrition* gets money from mega-giants General Foods, Quaker Oats, and Best Foods.[152] Other professional journals are sponsored by Slim-Fast Foods, the Sugar Association, Nestle/Carnation, and Coca-Cola, among others. Writes Schmid, "It is difficult to imagine why Coca-Cola would give money to a nutrition journal for any reason other than influencing the journal's content and policies."[153] The same could be said of the vast sums that the food giants give to the nutrition departments of universities. I'm going to assume that if you're reading this book, you understand how corporate money has essentially bought our entire political process. Ask yourself: why would our public health institutions be exempt?

That is the question which needs to be asked. Answering it would go a long way toward restoring our health, our communities, our democracy, and ultimately our one and only planet.

Gary Taubes's book *Good Calories, Bad Calories: Challenging the Conventional Wisdom on Diet, Weight Control, and Disease,* is a complete investigation into both the science and the politics of heart disease, cholesterol, and diet. He starts by analyzing the public myth-making in which the proponents of the Lipid Hypothesis have engaged:

> From the inception of the diet-heart hypothesis in the early 1950s, those who argued that dietary fat caused heart disease accumulated the evidential equivalent of a mythology to support their belief. These myths are still passed on faithfully to the present day. Two in particular provided the foundation on which the national policy of low-fat diets was constructed. One was Paul Dudley White's declaration that a "great epidemic" of heart disease had ravaged the country since World War II. The other could be called the story of *the changing American diet.* Together they told of how a nation turned away from cereals and grains to fat and red meat and paid the price in heart disease. The facts do not support these claims, but the myths served a purpose, and so they remained unquestioned.[154]

The story is that heart disease was rare at the beginning of the last century, increased in the 1920s, and exploded into the nation's number one killer by 1950. The facts, however, line up rather differently. What's missing from the standard narrative is a distinction between a disease's existence and its diagnosis. The first research paper on the diagnosis of CHD was written in 1912 by Dr. James Herrick. In 1918, he combined his protocol with the newly invented electrocardiogram, and the discipline of cardiology was born. Over the next ten years, the CHD diagnosis became widely enough accepted that doctors began to use it. Writes Taubes, "Between 1920 and 1930 ... physicians at New York's Presbyterian Hospital increased their diagnosis of coronary disease by 400 percent, whereas the hospital's pathology records indicated that the disease incidence remained constant during that period."[155]

The second factor casting doubt on a sudden CHD epidemic is the shift in life expectancy that took place in that same time period. Infectious diseases had been conquered by antibiotics and by better public health measures. In 1900, life expectancy was forty-eight; by 1950, it was sixty-seven. Vastly more people were living to an age where chronic diseases like heart disease and cancer would finally take their toll.[156]

The third factor was a revision in the International Classification of Diseases. The ICD is a comprehensive list of diseases used by physicians to identify the cause of death in the deceased. Arteriosclerotic heart disease was added in 1949. According to the American Heart Association, "Undoubtedly the wide use of the electrocardiogram in confirming clinical diagnosis and the inclusion in 1949 of Arteriosclerotic Heart Disease in the International List of Causes of Death play a role in what is often believed to be an actual increased 'prevalence' of this disease. Further, in one year, 1948 to 1949, the effect of this revision was to raise coronary disease death rates by about 20 percent for white males and about 35 percent for white females."[157] Common sense should tell you that CHD could not have risen 20 percent, let alone 35 percent, in one year. The World Health Organization admitted as much, commenting on the unlikelihood of a worldwide "epidemic" of CHD and pointing out that "much of the apparent increase in [coronary heart disease] mortality may simply be due to improvements in the quality of certification and more accurate diagnosis."[158]

Anthony Colpo clocks each successive change in the International Classification of Diseases—in 1929, 1948, 1968 and 1979—to another uptick in recorded CHD rates in the US. He writes:

> There are two possible explanations for the CHD mortality pattern shown ... The first one is that, during the twentieth century, coronary and non-coronary heart disease victims were doing an outstanding job of timing their deaths to cor-

respond precisely with the new ICD classification changes—a highly unlikely occurrence to say the least. The second and far more realistic explanation is simply that doctors were increasingly classifying victims into CHD- and non-CHD-related categories as the classifications became more specific, ECG machines became more widely used, and medical knowledge of heart disease increased. When the 1968 additions to the ICD criteria allowed doctors to assign the maximum possible percentage of heart disease deaths to the CHD category, CHD mortality hit its 'peak' then immediately began to decline in line with the overall heart disease trend.[159]

Researchers can calculate what are called "age-adjusted" death rates, that is, numbers that take into account any increase in overall life span. Obviously, this is necessary for any judgment about whether an apparent increase in some disease is real or merely a side effect of people living longer. For age-adjusted data, CHD hits its peak in 1968, but as noted, this was due to ICD classifications. Writes Colpo, "We therefore have every reason to believe that the historical age-adjusted peak for CHD occurred, not in 1968, but somewhere around 1950. As such, the true decline in CHD appears to have begun over a decade before the health establishment launched its campaign against saturated fat and cholesterol."[160]

The final factor in all these numbers—and it's a crucial factor—is the incidence of CHD versus the mortality from CHD. Mortality has been dropping for the simple reason that medical interventions have improved dramatically. The doctors in the Framingham study wrote that, as of 1990, "our data indicate that the decline in mortality was primarily the result of improved survival among persons with new cases of cardiovascular disease, rather than the result of a substantial decrease in the incidence of the disease."[161] Colpo credits "[a]mbulance and paramedic networks, the development of CPR techniques and electrical defibrillators, anti-clotting drugs, coronary care units, and campaigns to raise awareness of heart attack symptoms."[162] The authors of a ten-year study of CHD death rates, published in *The New England Journal of Medicine*, agreed.[163] Data from the American Heart Association make much the same point: between 1979 and 2003, the number of CHD in-patient procedures performed increased 470 percent. Cardiac catherizations were performed on over a million people in 2003.[164] Sources ranging from the Centers for Disease Control to the *British Medical Journal* all show that CHD is actually on the rise, even as heroic technologies save more lives.[165]

We've been doing what we've been endlessly badgered to do since the 1960s. We've eaten, according to the USDA, less fat, less meat, fewer eggs. Our dietary fat has fallen 10 percent, hypertension has dropped 40 percent and the number of us with chronically high cholesterol has declined 28 percent.[166] But we have not gotten any healthier. As Gary Taubes writes, "Indeed, if the last few decades were considered a test of the fat-cholesterol hypothesis of heart disease, the observation that the incidence of heart disease has not noticeably decreased could serve in any functioning scientific environment as compelling evidence that the hypothesis is wrong."[167]

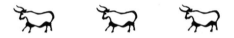

The myth told by the Lipid Hypothesizers has a second half. The rest of their story is that over the course of the twentieth century, the US American diet shifted from wholesome, virtuous grains to the gluttonous sins of meat and fat, with CHD as our just desserts. The numbers behind these supposed dietary patterns were originally assembled by Ancel Keys. The statistics he used, called "food disappearance data," are generated annually by the USDA. They "estimate how much we consume each year of any particular food, by calculating how much is produced nationwide, adding imports, deducting exports, and adjusting or estimating for wastage. The resulting numbers for per capita consumption are acknowledged to be, at best, rough estimates."[168]

The biggest problem with food disappearance data is that any foods that didn't enter the market couldn't be counted. Back when 50 percent of US Americans lived on farms, that would have includ-

ed lots of vegetables and fruits, and all kinds of animal products—
meat, eggs, dairy, and fish. The food disappearance data for the early
part of the last century shows that people in the US were consuming a diet based on grain products and potatoes because those
products were commodities that entered national and international
markets. The same would not be true of animal products until the
invention of factory farming and the death of the family farm. After
World War II, meat and other animal products assume a bigger proportion of the food disappearance data because those foods became
commodified as well. In other words, they were counted because
suddenly they *could* be counted, not because US Americans were
necessarily eating more of them.

These two myths—1. the sudden epidemic of heart disease,
caused by 2. an increase in US Americans' consumption of dietary
fat—are the scaffolding on which the proponents of the Lipid Hypothesis have built their paradigm. But if their structural support
amounts to nothing more than essentially bad record-keeping, why
have they been able to get this far? Why do they have a stranglehold
on the dietary wisdom and habits of the US? Surely, if they were so
completely off base, somebody would have said something.

In fact, there have been detractors all along, but to know about
them and their version of human biology, you'd have to read the
medical journals and attend professional conferences. The main de-
bates about the Lipid Hypothesis have happened largely out of the
public eye, even while vast sums of the public's money have been
spent, and a huge experiment on the public's health conducted. Tell
me, did you sign a check or a release form?

There has been another hypothesis to explain "heart disease,
diabetes, colorectal and breast cancer, tooth decay, and half-dozen
or so other chronic diseases."[169] Taubes names it the *carbohydrate
hypothesis*. This hypothesis began with years of observations by British doctors and missionaries who tagged along with the imperialists,
and found the same thing that Weston Price would discover: that
indigenous people eating their traditional foods were free from the
chronic illnesses that came to be known as the diseases of civilization. When such people moved to a town or had access to a trading

post, and began to eat sugar, flour, vegetable oil, and canned milk, the diseases followed. Writes Taubes:

> We have come to accept over the past few decades the hy-potheses—and that is what they are—that dietary fat, calories, fiber, and physical activity are the critical variables in obesity and leanness in health and disease. But the fact remains that, over those same decades, medical researchers have elucidated a web of physiological mechanisms and phenomena involv-ing the singular effect of carbohydrates on blood sugar and on insulin, and the effect of blood sugar and insulin, in turn, on cells, arteries, tissues, and other hormones, that explain the original observations and support this alternative hypothesis of chronic disease.[170]

The concept of "the diseases of civilization" was developed in the nineteenth century by a French doctor, Stanislaus Tanchou. His original research was on cancer, specifically its pattern of concentra-tion and proliferation. His research showed that cancer was an ur-ban phenomenon, not a rural one, and that it was spreading across Europe. He corresponded with doctors in Africa who witnessed the increase in cancer in populations that had been cancer-free, concomi-tant with their acculturation to European foods. My favorite Tanchou quote: "Cancer, like insanity, seems to increase with the progress of civilization."

Doctors across Africa submitted reports detailing essentially the same observations to publications like the *British Medical Journal* and *The Lancet*. And not just out of Africa. Articles and indeed entire books on the health of Native Americans from across North America appeared during the beginning of the twentieth century, drawing the same conclusions. Farther afield, British doctors reported from distant Fiji, where, among 120,000 Aborigines, there were exactly two reported cancer deaths.[171] This continued on into the mid-twen-tieth century. As late as 1952, an article out of Queen's University in Ontario opened with, "It is commonly stated that cancer does not occur in Eskimos, and to our knowledge no case has so far been reported."[172] Remember, those people were eating a diet that was 80 percent animal fat. Frederick Hoffman authored a book entitled, *The Mortality from Cancer Throughout the World* in 1915 and, in 1937, *Cancer and Diet*, the culmination of his life's work. He also founded the American Cancer Society. It was his conclusion that cancer, one of the prime diseases of civilization, is caused by the foods of civilization: "far-reaching changes in bodily functioning and metabolism are introduced which, extending over many years, are the causes or conditions predisposing to the development of malignant new growths, and in part at least explain the observed increase in the cancer death rate of practically all civilized and highly urbanized countries."[173]

British doctors gathered evidence from Asia as well. C.P. Donnison examined British Colonial Office medical reports, which compiled diagnoses from hospitals across the British empire. In his book *Civilization and Disease*, published in 1938, he wrote that many doctors encountered no diabetes in indigenous populations. But as the local people assimilated (whether forcibly or voluntarily) to civilized foods, "a great incidence is recorded."[174] At its 1907 conference, the British Medical Association organized a panel specifically on diabetes in the tropics. Both Indian and British doctors noted that "the Hindus, who were vegetarians, suffered more than the Christians or the Muslims, who weren't. And it was the Bengali ... whose daily sustenance ... was chiefly rice, flour, pulses and sugars who suffered the most—10 percent of 'Bengali gentlemen' were reportedly diabetic."[175]

Taubes writes that "the evidence continued to accumulate, virtually without counterargument."[176] By World War II, the concept of "protective foods" held sway: "fresh meat, fish, eggs, milk, fruits and vegetables."[177] The concept was formulated by Scottish nutritionist Robert McCarrison, based in part on his experience living in the Himalayas, which is about as isolated as it gets. There he found the usual: "I never saw a case of asthenic dyspepsia, of gastric or duodenal ulcer, of appendicitis, of mucous colitis, or of cancer..."[178] These comparisons between people eating their native diets versus the same people eating the foods of civilization produced the same conclusions through the 1960s: that a combination of diabetes, cancer, and heart disease would appear where previously there had been none.

The pieces of the disease puzzle started coming together as early as 1885, when a German researcher found that "sixty-two of seventy cancer patients were glucose-intolerant."[179] By the mid-1960s, scientists were observing that insulin stimulated malignancies to grow.[180] In 1967, Howard Temin, a Nobel prize-winning cancer researcher, found that without the presence of insulin, cancerous cells didn't grow. Other doctors noted the concurrence of diabetes and breast cancer. This was in 1956. And yet we've been told repeatedly to eat that high-carb diet, with its requisite insulin overload. "Low-fat, plant-based" is the endless round of rosaries that our public health institutions have to offer. In fact, prayer probably would be more effective—it could hardly be worse.

Another researcher, Robert Stout of Queen's University, Belfast, showed how insulin both increases the transfer of fats and cholesterol into the arterial walls and promotes the synthesis of fat and cholesterol within the arterial lining. In 1969, he co-authored a paper with diabetologist John Vallance-Owen, blaming "large quantities of refined carbohydrates" for all of it.[181] He would go on to show in 1975 that insulin triggers the growth of the smooth muscle cells of the arteries, the beginning of high blood pressure and arteriosclerosis.

Scientific studies had noted the concurrence of diabetes and CHD as early as 1929.[182] In the late 1940s, more research concluded that men with diabetes had twice the risk of CHD, and diabetic women three times the risk.[183] In 1961, researchers Pete Ahrens and Margaret Albrink both attended a meeting of the Association of American Physicians, reporting on research that linked elevated triglycerides with CHD. Triglycerides are created in the liver from dietary sugars. They both laid the blame for CHD squarely on a high-carbohydrate diet. By the early 1970s, Albrink's theory would be substantiated by researchers that included a future Nobel laureate.[184]

Of course, during this same time, Keys was publishing his Seven Countries Study and proposing fat as the cause of chronic diseases. John Yudkin, who created the first university nutrition department in Europe, directly challenged Keys's Lipid Hypothesis, publishing articles and books throughout the 1960s that focused on the causal relationship between the consumption of sugars, elevated insulin levels, and heart disease.[185] Protective foods didn't go down without a fight.

In 1973, George McGovern's Senate Select Committee on Nutrition and Human Needs convened its first hearing on chronic diseases and nutrition. Yudkin testified. So did Peter Cleave, Aharon Cohen, and George Campbell, along with other experts on diabetes and heart disease. There were plenty of highly credentialed people on hand to argue for the carbohydrate hypothesis, and argue they did.

As a side note, Gary Taubes points out that McGovern himself had spent a month at Nathan Pritikin's diet center.[186] By his own admission, McGovern was only able to stick to the low-fat Pritikin diet for a few days, yet Pritikin's ideas had made an impact on him. This disjuncture between theory and practice, between ideal and the experience of physical deprivation, is one I understand well, having stuck to a similar regime for rather longer than a few days myself. McGovern knew from his own attempt that the low-fat experiment wouldn't work: his own body had told him. Yet that wasn't the knowledge that won the day.

Despite the clear evidence that no scientific consensus had been reached, "The testimony would have little impact on the content of McGovern's *Dietary Goals for Americans*, in part because none of the staff members who organized the hearings would still be working for the committee three and a half years later, when the *Dietary Goals* would be drafted. Equally important, neither McGovern nor his congressional colleagues could reconcile what they were hearing from the assembled experts with what they had now come to believe about 'the nutritional evils of modern diets.'"[187]

In 1976, the committee heard two more days of experts, then turned the project over to Nick Mottern, a labor reporter hired as a writer by McGovern's staff. The final document he produced was based largely on the non-existent change in the US American diet, the mythic whole-grain diet of an earlier, healthier time. Mottern likened the food industry to the tobacco industry, except his critical perspective was selective: he attacked the meat and dairy associations, not the grain cartels.

The result, *Dietary Goals for Americans*, set in motion a vast sea change in the public's beliefs and behaviors. Writes Taubes, "*Dietary Goals* took a grab bag of ambiguous studies and speculation, acknowledged that the claims were scientifically contentious, and then officially bestowed on one interpretation the aura of established fact."[188]

At the press conference announcing the report's release, "[A]ll hell broke loose.... Practically nobody was in favor of the McGovern recommendations."[189] The committee had to hold eight more hearings to address the outcry. Another line of experts presented evidence against the Lipid Hypothesis. The American Medical Association submitted written testimony that stated "there is a potential for harmful effects for a radical long term dietary change as would occur through the adoption of the proposed nutritional goals."[190]

It didn't make any difference. Protective foods lost, and the Lipid Hypothesis won.

Or think of it this way. *Dietary Goals* was a predictable victory in a war that started ten thousand years ago. What really won were those annual grasses that had long since turned humans into mercenaries against the rest of the planet. We would now enshrine them like demi-gods, those whole grains and their sweet, opiate seductions, believing in their power to bestow health and long life, even while they slowly ate us alive.

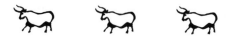

The research hasn't stopped. Not only does it keep disproving the Lipid Hypothesis, sometimes it even makes headlines. "Heart Attacks: A Test Collapses," stated the *Wall Street Journal* in October of 1982, reporting on the utter failure of MRFIT (Multiple Risk Factor Intervention Trial), a study sponsored by the National Heart, Lung and Blood Institute. It followed twelve thousand men for seven years. Half were counseled to stop smoking, eat a low-fat and low-cholesterol diet, and take high blood pressure medications if warranted—the multiple interventions referred to in the title. More of them died then the men who were left to eat and smoke as they pleased. In fact, more of them even died *from lung cancer* despite the fact that 21 percent of them quit smoking.[191]

And the data from Framingham keeps rolling in, though no one seems to notice what it says, sometimes the researchers least of all. As early as 1971, the data showed that the relationship between cholesterol levels and CHD for women under 50 was scant, and for women over 50 it was utterly absent. The doctors themselves said that cholesterol has "no predictive value." "This means," writes Gary Taubes, "women over fifty would have no reason to avoid fatty foods because lowering their cholesterol by doing so would not lower their risk of heart disease."[192]

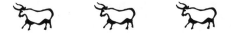

You want to read that again? No, first go get yourself a bowl full of something delicious with fat, something you've been denying yourself for the last twenty years. Whatever it is: go get some.

And while that delightful sense of well-being melts across your tongue and through your brain, read this: "Though women were clearly meant to adhere to the low-fat guidelines, they had not been included in any of the clinical trials. The evidence suggested that high cholesterol in women is not associated with more heart disease, as it might be in men, with the possible exception of women under fifty, in whom heart disease is exceedingly rare."[193]

Lick your spoons, gyrls. Then lick your bowls.

After twenty-four years of collecting data in Framingham, the researchers had found no correlation, let alone causality, between cholesterol levels and fatal heart attacks.[194]

Ready for seconds?

Let's look at the Nurses' Health Study out of Harvard. Eighty-nine thousand nurses have been followed since 1982. The first update came in 1987, in *The New England Journal of Medicine*: the *less* fat women ate, the *higher* their chance of breast cancer. In 1992, the next round was reported: again, lower fat, higher breast cancer risk. In 1999, another installment was published, and dietary fat was still *pro-*

tecting women from breast cancer. "For every 5 percent of saturated-fat calories that replaced carbohydrates in the diet, the risk of breast cancer decreased by 9 percent."[195] The National Cancer Institute found the same protection from breast cancer in saturated fat.[196]

Somewhere, a collection of French physicians and British Navy doctors are nodding their heads beside a Canadian dentist.

In 1997, the World Cancer Research Fund and the American Institute for Cancer Research, issued a 700-page report stating that there was neither "convincing" nor "probable" evidence to link high fat consumption to elevated cancer risk.[197] In 2006, the American Cancer Society said flat out that "there is little evidence that the total amount of fat consumed increases cancer risk."[198] Men, I think you can be excused to take your turn to hunt and gather for something satisfyingly fatty right about now.

And there's more. The National Institutes of Health spent $700 million on their Women's Health Initiative to track 49,000 women. In 2006, the results came back. The women who were convinced to eat the "healthy" diet—less fat, more whole grains and vegetables—had the same breast cancer risk as the control group. Comments Gary Taubes, "In the two decades since the NIH, the surgeon general, and the National Academy of Sciences first declared that all Americans should consume low-fat diets, the research has also failed to support the most critical aspect of this recommendation: that such diets will lead to a longer and healthier life. On the contrary, it has consistently indicated that these diets do more harm than good."[199]

And for those of you who resolutely refuse to even consider the above, I offer the following from the history of modern medicine: lobotomies, the Dalkon Shield, thalidomide, Electroshock Therapy, DES, Hormone Replacement Therapy, and Vioxx.

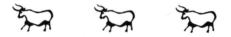

No discussion of vegetarian nutrition would be complete without a mention of soy. Soy has been heralded as a panacea for everything from hot flashes to world hunger. Big Agra has done its best to convince us that soy is healthy—ADM spent $4.7 million for airtime during *Meet the Press* and $4.3 million on *Face the Nation*[200]—even though no human beings have ever eaten the highly processed industrial products now being sold to the groovy, the smug, and the earnest across the US, and to their children, including their infants.

Soy started out as a legume that was rotated with other annual crops throughout Asia. Because it can fix nitrogen, soy was used as a green manure. The Chinese characters for barley, millet, rice, and wheat are pictures of the grains, because it's the edible parts that matter. The character for soy shows the roots, because it was grown as a cover crop, not a food.[201] Soy contains so many anti-nutrients that it isn't edible for humans without a lot of processing, substantially more than other seeds.

First of all, soy contains trypsin inhibitors. Trypsin, you'll remember, is a digestive enzyme produced in the pancreas. That's why eating soy causes gas, bloating, pain, and diarrhea. Fermenting soy will deactivate most of the trypsin inhibitors. In a study of fifty Asian cultures, the people that had found a way to disable the trypsin inhibitors were the only ones that considered soy edible.[202] Miso, which is highly fermented, entered the cuisine of Asia sometime between the second century BCE and the fourth century CE.[203] Tofu, which is not fermented, was invented in 164 BCE., and tempeh, which is fermented, was probably developed in the 1600s. Monks took to tofu because it helped them keep their vows of sexual abstinence: soy's phytoestrogens lower testosterone levels, and hence their libidos. "Except in areas of famine," writes soy expert Kaayla Daniel, "tofu was served as a condiment, consumed in small amounts, usually in fish broth, not as a main course."[204] The Chinese ate soy as a protein source only when they were starving—when they also ate their children.[205]

Fish broth is a key detail in the story of soy. If you make it past the intestinal distress caused by the trypsin inhibitors, the next problem with soy is the phytates. Phytates, remember, bind with minerals in your digestive tract, making them inaccessible. Soy has such a high level of phytates that no amount of soaking or fermenting will disable them all. You can see the wisdom in serving soy with fish broth, as the broth provides a large dose of minerals to counteract the phytates.

Soy is also a known goitrogen. Researchers have known since the 1930s that soy can suppress and permanently damage your thyroid if you eat enough of it. Kaayla Daniel writes,

> soy proponents scoff at the notion that soy causes thyroid problems because, they say, goiter is not a problem in Asia. In fact, the *New York Times* has reported an epidemic of cretinism in impoverished rural areas of China where iodine deficiency is widespread and poverty forces people to eat more soy than the small quantities that are the norm.... In Japan, where soy consumption is the highest of any country in Asia, thyroid disease is widespread. After all, Hashimoto's thyroiditis, the autoimmune form of hypothyroidism, was first detected in Japan, and the prevalence there of thyroid disease has motivated Japanese researchers to undertake important studies proving the adverse effects of soy foods on the thyroid gland.[206]

In 1980, government researchers in Britain identified soy-dependent vegans as a population at risk for thyroid disease. Since then, the British Committee on Toxicity (COT) has added to that list infants fed soy formula and adults using soy foods or soy supplements.[207] Researchers have known since the 1950s that soy foods cause thyroid damage, especially in infants. The insult is so strong that for some infants "hypothyroidism persists despite medication."[208] In a study done on healthy Japanese adults, thirty grams of soy for thirty days was enough to provoke thyroid disruptions.[209]

Thirty grams of soy was a snack when I was a vegan. And infants on soy formula are getting more than that. Britain's COT warned, "Even allowing for differences in absorption, the large differences in exposure [between soy and non-soy formula] would be expected to cause significant effects." [210] Here in the United States, the US Research Council observed, "The concentration of soy phytoestrogens that inhibit thyroid hormone biosynthesis is within the range of exposure of infants maintained on soy formula ... [T]hat concentration is six to eleven-fold higher than concentrations known to have a hormonal effects in adults."[211]

Another serious health consequence is hormonal disruption caused by soy's phytoestrogens. In a plant's array of potential weapons, phytoestrogens are essentially going for the throat in evolutionary terms. Trypsin inhibitors might make a hungry predator sick, but phytoestrogens make them unable to reproduce. Phytoestrogens are produced by more than three hundred plants, but soy is the only one that humans eat. Phytoestrogens have two routes to do their damage. First, they can lock onto estrogen receptors in the body, blocking true estrogen and other hormones. And second, they can also disrupt the body's production of estrogen.

If you believe that because a substance is "natural" it can't hurt you, get over it. Arsenic is natural. So, for that matter, is uranium. Phytoestrogens are powerful endocrine disruptors, especially in the amounts consumed by vegetarians. And remember the many happy endings provided by another estrogen mimic, diethylstilbestrol, aka DES.

Scientists have known that phytoestrogens disrupt mammalian reproduction since the 1940s, when sheep got "clover disease" from grazing pastures that had high levels of phytoestrogens in the plant mix. These phytoestrogens—formononetin, biochanin A, and genistein—caused "endometrial damage and cervical mucus changes associated with an inability to conceive."[212] In fact, phytoestrogens cause reproductive problems in "birds, cows, mice, cats and dogs as well as in humans."[213] The cheetahs at the Cincinnati Zoo had "liver disease and reproductive failure" because their food contained soy.

And in humans? This was information I had to brace myself to hear. Three months into my veganism, my menstruation had ground to a halt. The only thing the doctor could suggest was going on the Pill. Me? Hurt my body with pharmaceuticals? Invade my sacred wombmoon cycles with potent, potentially carcinogenic, and definitely misogynistic chemicals? She had to be joking.

Twenty years later, twenty years during which I'd had maybe fifty periods, I read that 60 grams of soy protein given for thirty days produced "significant biological effects," effects that lasted for three months after stopping the soy.[214] The women's cycles lengthened, mid-cycle levels of luteinizing hormone dropped 33 percent, and their follicle stimulating hormone dropped 53 percent. They were on their way to soy-induced infertility.

Sixty grams of soy protein—that's one cup of soy milk—contains 45 mg of isoflavones. One cup of tofu contains 56 mg. A mere half cup of dry roasted soy beans has 128 mg.[215] I'd been on the Pill all right, but the one made by Big Agra instead of Big Pharma.

There was more, lots more. Scientists from the Karolinska Institute in Sweden, in a study in *The Journal of Endocrinology*, wrote,

> these findings have raised concerns about human exposures to phytoestrogens. The widespread use of soya beans as a protein food source makes it important to determine possible physiological effects of equol [an isoflavone] in man [sic]. The contraceptive effect in animals suggests to us that it may be of interest to investigate the dietary habits and urinary excretion of equol in women with unexplained infertility or disorders of the menstrual cycle.[216]

In the 1970s WHO spent $5 million investigating potential "natural" contraceptives, in the hope of finding something safer than the pill. WHO researchers compiled data from around the globe, visiting indigenous cultures and gathering samples of plants that were used for contraceptives. Hundreds of samples were examined, including soy, flax, and red clover (one of the plants that causes "clover disease" in sheep). But the project ended unsuccessfully. "Not because 'natural' methods didn't work," explains Kaayla Daniel, "but because the side effects were similar to—and just as serious—as those of the birth control pill."[217]

Worse, in Italy, scientists found that isoflavone supplements were responsible for "significant increases in the occurrence of endometrial hyperplasia." This thickening of the uterine lining can be precancerous. These researchers called isoflavone supplements "potent drugs" and questioned "the long term safety of phytoestrogens with respect to the endometrium."[218]

I say "worse" because one of my oldest friends has endometriosis. We now know she got it from soy. The pain is debilitating, and there is no cure. It began a few months after she adopted soy as a dietary staple. Soon after the condition developed, she spent a year in Europe—a year with no soy milk, tofu, or fake meat. Miraculously, the endometriosis disappeared. On her return to the United States, and not knowing better, she went back to eating soy. The endometriosis returned with a vengeance. She loses a week out of every month to severe pain, all for the glory of soy. The only thing that's helped? Going on the Pill.[219]

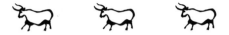

Here's a good example of how those with financial interests can twist research to suit their needs. The authors of the 60 gram study quoted above should have sounded the alarm about the harm phytoestrogens inflict. Instead, they hypothesized that eating soy could lower estrogen levels over the course of a woman's life, since women's menstrual cycles got longer on soy. This 100 percent speculation was then linked to the theory—a theory that hasn't been proven—that lower estrogen levels reduce the risk of breast cancer. So the researchers went so far as to propose soy isoflavones as a preventative agent against breast cancer. The main author, Aedin Cassidy, was given a job at Unilever, and the soy industry has been telling the media that soy prevents breast cancer ever since.[220]

Am I really the only person left in the US who thinks that interfering with the natural hormones of healthy women is self-evidently a bad idea? Didn't Hormone Replacement Therapy end up being the biggest cancer disaster of the century? Why are women's bodies always available for intervention, instead of defended on the basic principle of physical integrity and for the sake of those of us who live in one? Those are the questions I would like answered, especially by the next person who tries to feed me soy.

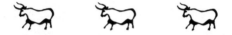

Soy also affects men's reproductive health. The male "clover disease" sheep had lowered sperm counts, infertility, and nipple discharge. Mouse sperm exposed to phytoestrogens were rendered incapable of fertilizing an egg. "Testosterone deprivation" has been triggered in lab animals by feeding them "isoflavone-rich diets."[221] Testosterone is a vital hormone needed for "growth, repair, red blood cell formation, sex drive and immune function."[222] So that's a whole other set of bodies that deserve to be left alone to take care of their own intricate life functions, without invasive disruptions that benefit only the bank ledgers of the powerful.

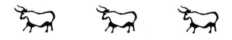

Never mind the enormous number of phytates leaching minerals from the body, and the dangers of disrupting women's natural levels of estrogen. Big Soya is also trying to prove that soy prevents osteoporosis. But so far, no good. As Kaayla Daniel reports, the results have been "disappointing, leading embarrassed researchers to explain that they haven't found a consistent bone-sparing effect because the dose must be either 'suboptimal' or 'excessive.' In other words, they *know* soy works, if they could only find the perfect dose, the perfect formula, the right age to initiate preventative treatment."[223]

Then there's what soy does to your brain. Dr. Lon R. White is a neuro-epidemiologist in Honolulu who used data from the Honolulu Heart Project to study over four thousand men and five hundred of their wives. Dr. White used cognitive testing, MRIs, and some autopsies to study nutrition and brain function. The data was unequivocal. Those who ate tofu at least twice a week had "accelerated brain aging, diminished cognitive ability, and were more than twice as likely to be clinically diagnosed with Alzheimer's disease."[224] There were enlarged ventricles on their MRIs, while the autopsied brains were atrophied. The researchers looked for every conceivable confounding factor—

age, weight, education, diet—and found none. In fact, "the more tofu eaten, the more cognitive impairment and/or brain atrophy."[225] According to a vegetarian bumper sticker, "There's no such thing as Mad Tofu Disease." You might want to rethink that—that's if you've got enough brain left to do the thinking.

Dr. White blames the isoflavones. Soy isoflavones can block tyrosine kinase, an enzyme needed by the hippocampus—the area of the brain responsible for memory and learning. Phytoestrogens also do more destruction here, lowering the concentrations of calcium-binding protein that protect the brain from neurodegenerative diseases. The phytoestrogen genistein in particular interferes with the brain's DNA synthesis, by reducing production of new brain cells and increasing cell death.[226] Here's a quote from Dr. White that someone should stamp on soy milk containers: "The bottom line is these are not nutrients. They are drugs."[227]

And I know this is purely anecdotal, but I've known a number of vegans with serious memory problems. Not people in their 70s, but people in their 20s. And I mean serious.

A friendly acquaintance asked me over for dinner. She ended her invitation with a directive to call her the night before the arranged date. I assumed it was so she could ask me about my menu preferences. When the day arrived, I made the call, and it was good that I followed though.

"Who?" she asked, friendly if confused.

"Lierre? Rhymes with Pierre? We talked at Jodi's party?"

"Oh, Lierre, right, with the chickens." That made her laugh. Then silence.

"You asked me to call?"

More silence. Okey-dokey.

"About tomorrow?"

Still more.

Damn the torpedoes. "You invited me over to dinner. You told me to call you to check in."

"Oh my god, I did, didn't I?" she bubbled.

"Listen, if tomorrow doesn't work—" I started bailing us both out as fast as I could.

"No, no, I want you to come. That's why I asked you to call. How about seven?"

We made small talk for a minute. She was friendly and funny. As I hung up I realized that she hadn't asked me about the menu. What was going on? Was she in an abusive relationship and needed help getting out? Was she considering some kind of political action and wanted my advice? Was she on drugs? I briefly considered a seething romantic interest but abandoned the idea—she'd hardly have forgotten who I was if she fancied herself in love. Oh, well.

Still confused, I arrived at her house at the appointed time. She took my coat, introduced me to her guinea pig, and led me into the kitchen.

"Do you want some tea?"

Tea? There was no dinner, and clearly no plan for one. Okay, sure, some tea. She put the cups on the table, beside a small tray of the usual choices: brown sugar, maple crystals, rice syrup, and stevia.

And then, "Milk? It's soy milk, I don't do dairy. I'm a vegan."

Yeah, no thanks.

"Oh, plain is fine," I replied, not wanting to jump into anything controversial as a guest at her table.

Suddenly her whole face lit up. "That's it! That's why I invited you over!"

I blinked, waiting.

"I heard you talking about soy! Does soy really cause memory problems?

I couldn't make it up if I tried.

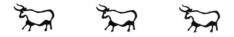

But the worst outrage is what soy does to babies. Soy-based infant formula "contains 130,000 times more isoflavones than human breast milk."[228] Does that scare you? That's nothing. Dr. Kenneth D.R. Setchell, of the Children's Hospital and Medical Center of Cincinnati, Ohio, concluded from his study that "the levels of phytoestrogens in soy formula are many times higher than in the breast milk of high soy consumers. Daily exposure of infants to isoflavones was four to eleven fold higher (on a body weight basis) than the dose that has hormonal effects in adults consuming soy foods."[229]

Now consider: DES is 100,000 times more potent than the phytoestrogens in soy foods. The soy industry wants you to stop right there, secure in the knowledge that they would never hurt your baby. I want you to keep reading. In 1985—that's over twenty years ago—Setchell wrote,

> while the potency of DES far exceeds that of either the endogenous estrogens or the phytoestrogens, the amounts consumed of the latter are significantly greater. The effects of plant estrogens in man [sic] should however be of some concern, particularly since it has been suggested that soya might be as beneficial a growth promoter as DES in animals. For example, the concentrations of phytoestrogens in soy, calculated to match 0.5 ppb of DES are well within the concentration range of commonly consumed soy products.[230]

Some animal studies show that phytoestrogens may cause *more* cancer than DES, depending on the stage of development at which the soy is consumed. Here's a quote from a researcher from the National Laboratory of Toxicology at the National Institute of Environmental Health Sciences: "The use of soy-based infant formulas in the absence of medical necessity and the marketing of soy products designed to appeal to children should be closely monitored."[231]

What happens to babies fed soy formula? First, soy formula provides 38 mg of isoflavones a day.[232] That's a hormone load equivalent to that of *three to five birth control pills* each and every day.[233] That number was derived from Swiss Federal Health Service data, data they published with warnings. Are you warned yet? Daniel Sheehan, who was a Senior Toxicologist at the FDA's National Center for Toxicological Research, thinks you should be. He says that infant soy formula is a "large, uncontrolled and basically unmonitored human infant experiment."[234]

Phytoestrogens can lock onto receptor sites for real hormones that the human body needs, like testosterone, estrogen, and progesterone. Effects range from structural changes in the brain to reproductive system and genital abnormalities. Researchers have had to come up with new terms to describe "the clusters of birth defects, the increased susceptibility to hormonal diseases and the altered behavioral patterns that occur in estrogenized boys."[235] They call it "Developmental Estrogenization Syndrome" or "Testicular Dysgenesis Syndrome." They could make things easy and call it Soy Syndrome. Hypospadias is one birth defect on the list. It's when the opening of the urethra is on the underside of the penis rather than at the tip. Boys with hypospadias often have undescended testicles and inguinal hernia as well. Over the last forty years, the United States and Europe have seen an alarming increase in hypospadias, especially in severe cases, which rules out better reporting as the explanation. And since it's not a global trend (the defect occurs overwhelmingly in rich nations), common sense rules out the agricultural and industrial chemicals the progressives would like to blame. Feel free to blame those for other horrors, like Pierre Robin syndrome and spina bifida, and then put your money on the phytoestrogens in soy: boys with hypospadias are *five times more likely* to have a vegetarian mom than an omnivorous one. The authors conclude that "a causal link is biologically feasible."[236]

What about girls? Right now, there is an epidemic of precocious female puberty in this country. One percent of US American girls have markers of puberty such as breast development or pubic hair *before age three*. I think that PCBs in plastic and endocrine disruptors in industrial chemicals are serious concerns, and I don't mean to let them off the hook. But precocious puberty breaks down by race: 14.7 percent of Caucasian girls show signs of puberty by age eight. But for African-American girls, that rate is *48.3 percent*. That's basically half. Please tell me your head is exploding with rage. No eight-year-old is emotionally prepared for puberty. And early puberty heralds a lifelong cascade of gynecological problems from amenorrhea to damaged follicles, along with "stunted growth, central nervous system disorders including headaches and seizures, reproductive complaints [and] behavioral problems."[237]

So where's the soy in this story? WIC (Women, Infants, and Children) is the federal food-distribution program for the poor. It gives out a lot of infant formula. WIC is required to get competitive bids from infant formula manufacturers in order to get it as cheaply as possible.

> WIC State agencies are required by law to have competitively-bid infant formula rebate contracts with infant formula manufacturers. This means a WIC State agency agrees to provide one brand of infant formula to its participants and in return receives money back, called a rebate, from the manufacturer for each can of infant formula that is purchased by WIC participants. As a result, WIC pays the lowest possible price for infant formula. The brand of infant formula provided by WIC varies from State agency to State agency, depending on which company has the rebate contract in a particular State.[238]

If you don't like the formula provided, you can change brands, but it usually takes a doctor's note. That is not an easy thing to get if you are a single woman with no transportation, small children, and a minimum-wage job with no benefits.

According to a Government Accountability Office (GAO) report, "Infants were least likely to be breastfed if their mothers were under 20 years old, not college-educated, unmarried [or] the infants were African-American."[239]

I could find no hard numbers on exactly how many African-American babies are getting soy formula. But the above isn't adding up to a pretty picture. The results—those 48 percent of Black girls entering puberty before they can join the Girls Scouts—speak for themselves, and they speak in a voice of outrage that no one hears. The cold contempt of racism, misogyny, and capitalism renders the dominant culture deaf. But the silence of progressives needs explaining.

Very successful campaigns have been waged against Nestle for its practices in Third World countries. Nestle's goal is, of course, to discourage breast-feeding and convince women that formula is better. But without the protective antibodies and nutrition of human breast milk, and with the water for mixing the formula carrying so many pathogens and parasites, babies die. According to UNICEF, a baby on formula in conditions of poverty and poor sanitation "is between six and 25 times more likely to die of diarrhea and four times more likely to die of pneumonia than a breastfed child."[240] Good people in the US and Europe petitioned and protested, and the struggle is ongoing. It's a righteous and honorable campaign.[241] My question is why no one cares about the vulnerable babies in the US. Forty-eight percent is one of those numbers that's almost too large for human speech to bear, or not if speech is still a conduit for the heart. But the Left is not taking this up. The only time these statistics are mentioned is when the culprits named are PCBs and a chemical company.[242]

Progressives are not looking at soy as a danger, a perpetrator stealing the childhoods of the vulnerable. They need soy to be a part of the solution, an integral piece of the Eco-Kingdom Come. Soy means that no one anywhere has to use animals for meat or milk: the lion shall lie down with the lamb. Soy means that all those wasted acres can feed people instead of beef cows. Soy heralds the low-fat paradise where our self-denial is our redemption, where we will be tempted no more by the Satan of bodily hungers and pleasures. We have sinned the sin of gluttony; the world is straining under our greed; and soy is our sacrament, it's here in your grocer's freezer, in cartons, in entrees, in our daily bread, in fact it's in 70 percent of all food now, the heavenly host that will redeem us. We are the Chosen Ones, and we know it, filling our carts with aseptic boxes and clean, light burgers. Even our snacks come consecrated, soy chips and nuts and desserts. Soy is great, soy is good. Only a heretic would question soy and the world to come.

Will it help if I tell you that Solae—which produces ingredients for soy foods like Gardenburgers, Mori-Nu, and Yves Veggie Cuisine—is owned by DuPont? You know they're poisoning the world.

Why do you trust them suddenly to manufacture (and it is manufacturing, not growing) your food?

This is what you're eating when you eat soy: an industrial waste product. Soy as it grows in the field is not actually a low-fat paragon. It's about 30 percent fat. Once upon a time it was grown for its oil—not because people ate it, but because it was used for paint and glue. In 1913, the USDA listed soy as an industrial material, not as a food.[243] Extracting the oil from soy leaves a defatted mass of protein. The question for industrial agriculture has been what to do with it. In 1975, a smart soy marketer said, "The quickest way to gain product acceptability in the less affluent society ... is to have the product consumed on its own merit in a more affluent society."[244]

Thirty years and millions of marketing dollars later, the affluent are happy to oblige. Soybean growers are required to pay 0.5 to 1 percent of their profits to the industry council, United Soybean. United Soybean spends $80 million every year in marketing. That's a lot of Caribbean vacations for the advertising and public-relations firms who've sold the affluent on the benefits of soy. And the affluent are buying. Soy milk alone went from $600 million in 2001 to over $892 million by 2006[245] on the strength of glossy, green ads in *Yoga, Self, Mother Jones,* and *Utne Reader.* The toned, the narcissistic, and the liberal have been converted, and their dollars follow their faith. Nobody thinks of soy as cheap filler for industrial food anymore. And like most faith-based beliefs, the belief in soy the Redeemer, the Prince of Peace, cannot survive rational scrutiny.

Soy milk is made by first soaking beans in an alkaline solution and then cooking them under pressure. Both the high pH and the pressure damage important nutrients in the beans, like the vitamins, the sulfur-based amino acids and especially the lysine. In the process, a toxin called lysinoalanine can be created. Manufacturers are also up against lipoxygenase, an enzyme in soy which oxidizes its polyunsaturated fats. It's these rancid oils that are largely responsible for the unpleasant odor and taste of soy milk. The bigger manufacturers deodorize the soy milk using "extremely high temperatures in the presence of a strong vacuum,"[246] the same industrial technique that's used in manufacturing vegetable oils. This process is only partially successful. To render the results palatable, sweeteners and flavorings have to be added, ranging from one teaspoon to one tablespoon of sugar per eight ounces. Writes Kaayla Daniel:

> Eliminating the aftertaste is a particularly challenging task. The undesirable sour, bitter and astringent characteristics come from oxidized phospholipids (rancid lecithin), oxidized fatty acids (rancid soy oil), the antinutrients called saponins, and the soy estrogens known as isoflavones. The last are so bitter and astringent that they produce dry mouth. This has put the soy industry into a quandary. The only way it can make its soy milk please consumers is to remove some of the very toxins that it has assiduously promoted as beneficial for preventing cancer and lowering cholesterol.[247]

What results from this process has to be fortified, usually by adding calcium and vitamin D2. D2 is a synthetic form of vitamin D which may cause "hyperactivity, coronary heart disease and allergic reactions."[248] The "milk" also has to be emulsified and stabilized, to keep all these substances hanging together. Titanium oxide—a mineral pigment used in white paint—has been used for this purpose. "Those who did not shake the containers thoroughly enough often found watery soy milk with lumps of white glop at the bottom," reminds Kaayla Daniel.[249] I can remember the exact taste and texture of that glop.

Soy cheese usually starts with hydrogenated oils as a base. There is no safe level of consumption of hydrogenated oils. Soy burgers, hot dogs, bacon and other faux meat products are made from textured soy protein (TSP), soy protein concentrate (SPC), and soy protein isolate (SPI). These are seriously scary industrial products. TSP, which is often sold plain in bulk bins at food co-ops, is made from soy flour. First the flour is defatted, using high temperatures and a hexane solution. The resulting paste is pushed through an extruder "under conditions of such extreme heat and pressure that the very structure of the soy protein is changed."[250] Colors, flavorings, and sweeteners are then added. The high heat and pressure destroy some of soy's antinutrients, but they also damage the amino acids beyond recognition while producing some frightening toxins.

Soy protein concentrate is manufactured by "precipitating the solids with aqueous acid, aqueous alcohol, moist heat and/or organic solvents."[251] SPI is ubiquitous in the US American food supply, added to everything from breakfast bars to hot dogs. It's also the main ingredient in soy-based infant formula. Writes Kaayla Daniel, "[T]he basic procedure begins with a defatted soybean meal, which is mixed with a caustic alkaline solution to remove the fiber, then washed in an acid solution to precipitate out the protein. The protein curds are then dipped into yet another alkaline solution and spray dried at extremely high temperatures."[252] Some amino acids are destroyed; others are rendered toxic and carcinogenic. The minerals in SPI are harder to utilize and the poor experimental animals fed soy protein isolate end up with deficiencies of "calcium, magnesium, manganese, molybdenum, copper, iron and especially zinc."[253] To turn the result into something a person might consider eating, the SPI has to be further processed using an alkaline solution with a pH above 10, more pressure and heat extrusion, and an acid bath, then mixed with the various binders, gums, fats, flavors, and sweeteners. Hungry yet? According to Daniel, "Spun soy protein fibers are not much different from plastic fibers; both are difficult to digest, have a 'scouring effect' on the GI tract and cause marked amounts of flatulence."[254]

The two main toxins produced in this process are nitrosamine and lysinoalanine. Liver damage from nitrosamines was established in 1937, and scientists have known for fifty years that nitrosamines are both carcinogenic and mutagenic.[255]

Lysinoalanine toxicity varies among test animals, but problems range from kidney damage to mineral deficiencies. I'm probably correct in assuming that you wouldn't buy shampoo that was tested on animals. But your basic food staples? And why would anyone knowingly eat food—"food"—that had to be so tested?

In the 1970s, SPI was ruled safe for use as *an ingredient in cardboard*. Researchers were worried that nitrosamine and lysinoalanine might leach from the cardboard container into food. Forty years later, the cardboard is safer to eat than the food. One hundred grams of soy protein a day could mean consuming *thirty-five times* the levels of nitrosamine considered safe.[256]

Not only does the manufacture of SPI create toxins, but the alkaline solutions, hot temperatures, and high pressure also destroy the structure of some of the amino acids, rendering them useless. Alkaline baths in particular result in low iron levels, and dramatically increase copper levels. Compromised zinc-copper ratios may be a causative factor in a range of mental illnesses, including depression, anxiety, and anorexia and in diseases like diabetes and rheumatoid arthritis.[257]

Dr. Ghulam Sarwar of Health Canada's Nutrition Research Division, states bluntly, "The data suggests that LAL (lysinoalanine), an unnatural amino acid derivative formed during processing of foods, may produce adverse effects on growth, protein digestibility, protein quality and mineral bioavailability and utilization. The antinutritional effects of LAL may be more pronounced in sole-source foods such as infant formulas and formulated liquid diets which have been reported to contain significant amounts (up to 2400 ppm of LAL in the protein) of LAL."[258]

There's more, lots more. There's excitotoxins, heterocyclic amines, furanones, chloropropanols, and hexanes. Don't know what they are? Then don't eat them. More importantly, don't let your children eat them.

But, again, don't they eat soy in Asia? Yes, but it's eaten in small amounts, basically as a condiment. Numbers vary, but here are some examples. The China-Cornell-Oxford study recorded the food intake of 6,500 Chinese adults. On average, 12 grams of legumes were eaten daily; one-third was soy. The math is easy: 4 grams a day.[259] One organization put Japanese consumption at 18 grams a day, which is a rounded tablespoon. Mark Messina, a champion of soy, thinks the Japanese eat 8.6 grams a day.[260] Another source puts soy at 1.5 percent of calories consumed by the Japanese—and pork, with its vitamin D rich-fat, at 65 percent.[261]

The long-lived Okinawans? Estimates vary on how much soy is in their diet. But they do eat 100 grams of both pork and fish every day.[262] And the kind of soy they eat is as important as how much. The highly fermented forms deactivate some of the antinutrients, especially when eaten along with mineral-rich, thyroid-supportive seafood and fish broth. They're not eating anything made by DuPont.

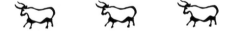

Read Kaayla Daniel's book, *The Whole Soy Story*, before you take another bite. Daniel writes that soy has caused "infertility, miscarriages, birth defects, decreased libido, anxiety, social isolation, aggression and other behavioral disorders in all animal species tested."[263]

Or listen to the Swiss Federal Office of Health: "Soya-based infant feeding should be used *only* when there is a clear medical indication. It should *never* be used for ecological or ideological reasons such as strict vegetarianism."[264]

In France, manufacturers will soon be required to remove the phytoestrogens in infant formula and to put warning labels on soy foods. In Israel, the health minister declared that infants should not be given soy formula, and that adults should be aware of the *increased* risk of breast cancer from eating soy. The New Zealand government has also issued a warning about soy formula for infants. Remember that soy has had a harmful effect on every test animal that has had the misfortune to be so used. Dr. Richard Sharpe, Director of the Medical Research Centre for Reproductive Biology in Edinburgh, Scotland, has this to say: "I've seen numerous studies showing what soy does to female animals. Until I have reassurance that it doesn't have this effect on humans, I will not give soy to my children."[265] The Federal Institute for Risk Assessment in Berlin, Gemany, has warned against feeding soy to babies unless under strict medical supervision, citing both the estrogenic isoflavones and the phytates. They also issued a warning about soy to adults: "When administered at high doses in isolated or fortified form, isoflavones impair the functioning of the thyroid gland and can change mammary gland tissue."[266]

And in the United States? Cornell University's Program of Breast Cancer and Environmental Risk Factors warned women at risk for breast cancer to avoid eating soy. After endorsing soy in 1999, the nutrition committee of the American Heart Association did a turn-around in 2006, announcing that soy confers no benefit and that the organization "therefore does not recommend isoflavone supplements in food or pills."[267] And while it's true that the FDA has endorsed soy as "heart healthy," that endorsement was based on a meta-analysis of studies on soy and heart disease—a meta-analysis paid for by PTI (Protein Technologies International, which is partly owned by Du-Pont).[268]

One soy researcher admitted publicly in 2001 that:

> Clinical work is driven by the idea that the isoflavone levels of Asians were extremely high and that low incidences of hormonal disease was due to high circulating levels of these compounds. If we look at a new cohort study in Japan, we see an average intake of 6-8 g per day. If you do rough calcula-tions as I did, I would estimate that the approximate levels of isoflavones were 15-30 mg per day and not, as I must admit, I rather erroneously stated in 1984. We thought perhaps then that it was 150-200 mg. We were going on very little data at the time..."[269]

Very little data: remember those three words.

Right now, there's a 30 percent limit on soy products in school lunches. The soy industry has paid public relations firm Norman Roberts Associates to help them get more soy into more school cafete-rias. In response to their pressure, the USDA offered to eliminate the 30 percent limit entirely. If that happens, public-school children—es-pecially the twenty-six million who qualify for free lunch programs, the ones who have probably already exceeded multiple lifetimes' worth of phytoestrogens, goitrogens, and carcinogens in their free infant formula—will once again become a dumping ground for Big Agra's industrial waste products. An entire generation of poor kids could be at risk. Will we—the people who lay claim to justice, com-passion, human rights—cling to our ideologies? Or will we fight for those kids?

Let's talk about vegetarian nutrition and eating disorders. Somewhere between 30 and 50 percent of the girls and women seeking treatment for anorexia and bulimia are vegetarian. About a third of the patients at the eating disorders program at Bloomington Hospital in Bloomington, Indiana, are vegetarian. At the Harvard Eating Disorder Clinic it's the same. Sheri Weitz, a nutrition therapist for the Radder Institute in Los Angeles has fully half her clients identifying as vegetarian.[270]

For years I struggled to understand why. Why would women who cared about animals and the earth be so vulnerable to eating disorders? I went looking for answers in social psychology, and I never found any. It turns out there is an explanation, but it's not political. It's biochemical. Vegetarian diets are typically low in tryptophan, which is the precursor for serotonin. Writes Julia Ross, "Over and over, studies have shown that removing tryptophan from our diet lowers serotonin and increases depression (including winter depression), insomnia, panic, and anger, and also triggers bulimia and chemical dependency."[271]

The vegetarian women and girls who turn up at eating disorder clinics in such huge numbers didn't start as anorexics who just happened to choose a vegetarian diet. It was the other way around. They started by choosing vegetarianism, and the lack of tryptophan triggered an eating disorder. Zinc deficiency also plays a role in mood disorders and obsessive compulsive behavior, including eating disorders. And a zinc deficiency is easy to court as a vegetarian.

The overlap in my life is a perfect 100. Everyone I've known with an eating disorder has been a vegetarian—and that includes two anorexic men, who were both vegans. Do I think eating disorders are that simple? Yes and no. The original impulse may be the compulsory self-hatred that this current version of patriarchy inflicts on women and girls. In male-dominated societies, including this one, the female body is always out of control, always needs to be constrained and punished. Right now those constraints are about size. "A cultural fixation on female thinness is not an obsession about female beauty but an obsession about female obedience," wrote Naomi Wolf in *The Beauty Myth*.[272]

The female body doesn't naturally obey. It naturally stores fat for gestation, to build the next generation. We have a word in English, *gaucy*, which means "fat and comely"—clearly a word that's fallen into disuse, although I'm doing my personal best to revive it. But the word's existence points to the fact that female fat is not universally despised; even in our culture there was once literally more room for women's bodies. But it takes the average woman twenty seconds of looking at fashion magazines to feel shame, guilt, and self-loathing. The vast majority of us are constantly dieting. Writes Marya Hornbacher in her book *Wasted: A Memoir of Anorexia and Bulimia*:

> In the hospital, women shriek and holler about how much they're eating: "But NO ONE eats this much!" Unfortunately, that has some truth to it. There are precious few women who eat normally. You get out of the hospital, look around at what other people are eating, and realize the nice little meal plan you're on—though you need it to stay healthy—is not the norm.[273]

And dieting produces its own biochemistry. Specifically, the lack of tryptophan, zinc, and niacin can trigger a full-blown eating disorder. Adolescents are most vulnerable because their bodies and brains are still growing and have higher nutritional needs. Julia Ross has treated teenage girls who became anorexic while on their very first diet. The precipitating incident is, essentially, living in this female-hating culture. What begins as simple dieting ends in an addictive cycle of either binging and purging or plain starvation. She writes:

> Why is it so easy to become bulimic? One reason is that both binging and vomiting can trigger waves of the potent brain chemicals—the endorphins. The release of these natural heroin-like brain chemicals helps establish the powerful compulsions that bulimics are helpless to fight. When we develop

false ideas about what we 'should' weigh and begin dieting, we open ourselves up to the possibility of developing an eating disorder.[274]

Ross identifies the nutritional deficiencies that cause the biochemistry of anorexia. Most important is the lack of tryptophan. Tryptophan is the amino acid that our brains use to make serotonin, which is the neurotransmitter that provides us with our basic feelings of well-being and self-esteem. As the dieter deprives herself of food, her serotonin levels drop, leaving her with a lessened sense of basic well-being and with more compulsions. "Tragically," writes Ross, "they [teenage girls] don't know that they will never be thin enough to satisfy their starving minds. Extreme dieting is actually the worst way to try to raise self-esteem, because the brain can only deteriorate further and become more self critical as it starves."[275]

The body's store of thiamine (B1) quickly runs low on a diet, and thiamine deficiency triggers a loss of appetite. "Suddenly dieting becomes easy," explains Ross. "You aren't fighting a normal appetite anymore. You lost it when you lost too much vitamin B-1 from dieting."[276]

As for zinc, it's a mineral that's not always easy to come by. Red meat and egg yolks are the best sources, but dieters and vegans both are going to avoid those. Zinc deficiency causes loss of both taste and of appetite, rendering food completely unappealing to the sufferer. Julia Ross reports that a five-year study "showed an astounding 85 percent recovery rate for anorexics patients given zinc supplementation."[277]

So here's how the cycle works. Going vegetarian or going on a diet causes a tryptophan deficiency, which causes serotonin levels to drop. As they drop,

you may become obsessed by thoughts you can't turn off or behaviors you can't stop. Once this rigid behavior pattern emerges in the course of dieting, the predisposition to eating disorders is complete. Just as some low-serotonin obsessive-compulsives wash their hands fifty times a day, some young dieters may begin to practice a constant, involuntary vigilance regarding food and the perfect body. They become obsessed with calorie counting, with how ugly they are, and on how to eat less and less. As they eat less, their serotonin levels fall farther, increasing dieters' obsession with undereating. As their zinc and B vitamin levels drop low as well, their appetite is lost. This can be the perfect biochemical set up for anorexia.... [J]ust as vitamin C deficiency (scurvy) results in an outbreak of red spots, so does tryptophan (and serotonin) deficiency result in an outbreak of the obsessive compulsive behavior we call 'control.' There may be psychological elements in the picture, too, but a low serotonin brain is ill-equipped to resolve them.[278]

The final nail in the coffin—and I don't mean that as a joke—is that both the starvation of anorexics and the binging-purging of bulimics can trigger a huge release of endorphins. That endorphin hit can be quite literally addictive. We know this because when anorexics and bulimics are given the same drugs that prevent opiates from affecting the brains of heroin addicts, they, too, go into withdrawal. Ross writes:

> Like laboratory monkeys who pull the lever that gives them heroin in preference to food or drink until they die, an anorectic will ferociously defend her refusal to eat for powerful biochemical reasons. Bulimics binge and refuse to keep food down with a similar ferocity for the same reasons. This obsessive behavior is actually caused by nutritional deficiencies—which, thankfully, we now know how to address.[279]

Even years into their recovery, all it takes is a few hours of tryptophan depletion to send some bulimics into relapse. That's one, maybe two skipped or inadequate meals. The same thing is true for depressives: even a few hours with not enough tryptophan and depression stirs in its lair.[280] I know, because I am what that beast will eat if it wakes completely. So, no, I can't come to your weekend conference, your groovy retreat, with its righteous, light meals of rice cakes and fruit, not if I can't bring my own food. I lost twenty years to depression: most of my youth. The world has color now, even beauty, and I am grateful every day. I'm the one that got away. But my brain, and the world it makes possible to me, needs to be fed. It's simple: I need at least three ounces of real protein in the morning or by noon the world begins to turn to sharp cliffs of anxiety and despair. Beyond that is the endless fall into gray nothing. And I'm not going back to that.

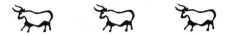

This is what I did to myself: I destroyed my body, the only one I was given. I want to say it was an honest attempt at an honorable life, because it was, but "honest" leaves out too much. I read survivor narratives of eating disorders, and I recognize way more than I want to. Is it because we inhabit the same brain, the vegans and the anorexics? A brain deprived of nutrients, its synapses in shreds, a brain that's literally falling to pieces? Anorexics have holes in their brains; so do eaters of soy. I try to explain to a friend how hard, how gruesome, this book has been to write. "Veganism," I quip, "is one part cult, one part eating disorder." I hear those words and I wish they weren't true because of what they mean about me.

Or I go out to lunch with a political caucus. There are two vegans at our table. I watch them order, listen to their voices as they talk to the waiter. I see the ferocity, the fear. Oh, I remember. They might eat some dreaded substance by mistake, just like the anorexics. As Hornbacher reminds us,

> [r]emember, anorexics do eat. We have systems of eating that develop almost unconsciously. By the time we realize we've been running our lives with an iron system of numbers and rules, the system has begun to rule us. There are systems of Safe Foods, foods not imbued, or less imbued, with monsters and devils and dangers. These are usually "pure" foods, less

likely to taint the soul with such sins as fat, or sugar, or an excess of calories. Consider the advertisements for food, the religious lexicon of eating: "Sinfully rich," intones the silky voiced announcer, "indulge yourself," she says, "guilt-free." Not complex foods that would send the mind spinning in a tornado of possible pitfalls contained in a given food—a possible miscalculation of calories, a loss of certainty about your control over chaos, your control over self. The horrible possibility that you are taking more than you deserve.[281]

When my body began to fall apart, why didn't I stop? Was it because I didn't know? It's not like you eat one vegan meal and the next day you're toast. It happened slowly. And no one out there was warning me. All the nutritional advice du jour was low-fat this and plant-based that. No doctor ever asked about my diet. Not one.

Would a normal person have stopped hurting herself? That's what I need to know. Should it have been self-evident that I was damaging my body? Not too long ago, I had a conversation with someone half my age.

"Oh, vegan," she said. "I was vegan for two weeks when I was seventeen. I was so exhausted I couldn't tie my shoes. So I went out for a burger and I felt *great*," she laughed, the way people laugh when they've got a funny story and they're happy to be alive.

Two weeks? She knew at two weeks what took me twenty years to figure out?

At some point the scale tips from honorable to fanatic. Dr. Steven Bratman has coined the term *orthorexia nervosa*, a pathological fixation on eating proper food.[282] One recovering vegan writes of being

swallowed up by alternative dietary theories often infested by mesmerizing double-think that effectively insulates the individual from any possible counterargument ... Emotional 'certainty' shuts down one's ability to rationally assess symptoms. By the time this happens, though, people have been so thoroughly convinced of the entire [raw vegan] dietary system

... that they are now psychologically invested in the 'rightness' of everything about the ... system, and cannot believe there could be any shortcomings in it, since it seems so internally self-consistent logically.[283]

And at some point it's the biochemistry speaking. The purity obsessions, the food control, the binges, the anxiety, the depression, the flares of rage, the impossible demands. Vegans, you have a reputation for a reason. Without protein and fat, the brain is reduced to rigidity and obsession. Yes, I know that animals are being tortured and the planet is dying. I know it's an emergency. I know it as much as you do, okay? But you don't have to kill yourselves or each other.

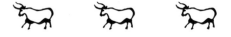

No one told me. No one told me that life is only possible through death, that our bodies are a gift from the world, and that our final gift is to feed each other. No one told me that soil was the beginning place, made of a million tiny creatures who turned this bare rock into a cradle. No one told me about my real parents; I learned about photosynthesis in seventh grade, but no one told me it was a lullaby.

And no one told me that civilization was a war, that agriculture was the end of the world. I was told that eating those foods, those annual monocrops, would save the world. So I ate. I was always hungry, but I believed that righteousness and justice would have to be nourishment. I made it be true. Body and brain wore down, day by day. To the very last hour of my vegan life, I made it be true.

On that last day, I went to see a Chi Gong master. He had cured the incurable. He learned Chi Gong as a boy in China, emigrated to the US, endured a life of hardship. He had very kind eyes. He took my pulses, which is the basic diagnostic tool of Chinese medicine. The practitioner reads the chi, the life force, that animates the body with different vital energies, to see where the patient needs help.

Or, he tried to take my pulses. Then he stared at me, half in awe, half in horror.

"There's nothing here," he said, unbelieving. "You have no chi."

"What, am I dead?" I joked, only he didn't laugh.

"You are so tired," he said.

Unspeakably. And I also refused to say it. I couldn't.

"Your menstrual cycle?" he asked.

"Infrequent." If ever, I could have added.

"And this problem with your spine," he said. He put his hands over my body and it was like nothing I've ever felt. He was a sieve, and my body was water. From my head down, slowly down, he somehow filtered through my spine. He hit the beginning of the degenerating area.

"Oh," he said. Down, and still down, to the part that aches like shrapnel every waking minute. Grade Four derangement, said the priests of radiology, reading the entrails of my bones.

"Oh," he said again. It was the most compassionate syllable I'd ever heard. "You should have come to me a long time ago."

And I knew I would leave there uncured. He couldn't help me. Too late.

"What do you eat?" he asked, and my heart snapped to alert.

"I don't eat ..." I began, but words were getting harder to find. I knew. I knew what was coming. I knew what I was going to have to face. "No animal products."

"No meat? No chicken? No fish?" he repeated.

I nodded. I didn't want to cry.

"No," he said, gently and absolutely. "This you cannot do."

I started crying.

"You have some religious belief?" he asked kindly.

"I—I—" I stammered. Everything was coming apart. I lived in a universe where no animals ever died for me, where my food was sustainable, where no one starved because of my unthinking cruelty or greed. None of that was true, of course, but I didn't know that then. All I knew was that those beliefs were the structural members of my identity, my daily actions, my political program, my relationship to the cosmos. And I was going to have to abandon everything, and live in a universe I found repellent.

"I don't want to hurt any animals," I begged like a child.

"The big fish eat the little fish," he offered sympathetically.

"But I'm not a fish," I wailed.

He shrugged to say, yes, you are, we all are. But I wasn't ready to know that. All I knew was before and after, and I stood on the exact point of my life's continental divide. He knew the truth of me: I was a corpse that only moved through sheer stubborn will. My body's basic structure was caving in slowly. I was so cold my hands and feet ached nine months of the year. And I could not have produced a baby if the entire species depended on it.

He did what he could for thirty minutes, and when I left, I didn't go home. I went to the store. The line wasn't long—I had to measure upright tasks in sixty second increments then—one minute to shop, plus a two-minute line plus sitting five minutes to get home. I could do it. I had to. I had to get this over with.

In a nihilistic way it was win-win. If I tried it and nothing happened, I'd never have to do it again. If I tried it and he was right, well, then I would feel better and ... and I would feel better and deal with the consequences to my identity and my world.

I had been a vegan over half my life. I bought a can of tuna fish.

I sat at my kitchen table with a plastic fork. I didn't use my silverware or my dishes. I opened the can. How could I actually do this? I broke it down into the tiniest steps. Pick up the fork. Put the fork in the tuna. I was so desperate. Pain was the inhabitant of my body, and I was only the shadow it cast. Lift the fork toward you. I had come to the end. Open your mouth. And I was so, so tired.

I ate it.

I don't know how to describe what happened next. "I felt like I was coming out of a coma," one ex-vegan told me. "It was like being plugged into a low-voltage battery," another friend said. I could feel every cell in my body—literally, every cell—pulsing. And finally, finally being fed.

Oh, god, I thought: *this is what it feels like to be alive.*

I put my head down and sobbed.

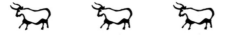

I cried every day for three weeks. And I ate meat every day. I had to lie down afterward, the recharge was so intense. Eventually it faded. Eventually I stopped crying. Eventually I told my friends. Some of them confessed that they too had started eating meat, or in fact had never really stopped. And some of them I lost.

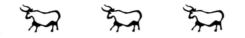

This is what will happen if you eat vegetarian, especially if you go vegan, for any length of time. Maybe not all of these things, but some of them. You will wear out your insulin receptors. The human body was never meant to absorb that amount of sugar. You can call it "complex carbohydrates" if you want, but it's sugar. The hypoglycemia will make you shake, sweat, and crave, god, those cravings. You'll feel like you're going to die if you don't put food in your mouth every three hours, every two hours, then thirty minutes after you eat. Hypoglycemia is its own emotional hell: the sudden weepiness, the temper fits, the instability. It's inexplicable when you're living it, and you also think it's normal, just life. It'll get worse every year. And yes, obviously you could do this to yourself as an omnivore. The standard US American diet contains vast quantities of sugar, with or without the meat. But it's hard to avoid as a vegetarian unless you live on eggs and cottage cheese, and impossible to avoid as a vegan.

You will destroy your bones and joints. You won't get enough minerals; unless you pretreat every seed (grains, nuts, beans), the phytates will bind with what few minerals you are ingesting; and you won't have enough dietary fat to absorb whatever is left. And you won't have enough vitamin D to build bone matrix, or enough zinc to build collagen.

The polyunsaturated fats, unstable and rancid, will wreck your blood vessels, your heart. Without protective saturated fats, adequate protein, and enough vitamin D, you will be at tremendous risk for cancer, especially the kinds that kill. Remember that hunter-gatherers don't get cancer. Remember who does.

The high omega-6s (and the nonexistent omega-3s) will create inflammation everywhere. Your joints, your blood vessels, your gut, your liver, your nerves, your brain are all potential victims. Maybe you'll get fibromyalgia. Maybe you'll get Alzheimer's. Maybe you'll have unnamed low-level pain where everything aches and you hate to be touched or jostled. It's because everything's inflamed.

On the low-fat and vegan versions especially, you'll have menstrual problems, fertility problems. Jorge Chavarro and his colleagues at the Department of Nutrition at Harvard found that women who ate two or more servings a day of low-fat instead of full-fat dairy foods increased their risk of ovulation-related infertility by more than four-fifths. That's 85 percent.[284] You'll get fibroids, cysts, endometriosis. If you do manage to have a baby, you're *five times* as likely to have a child with birth defects.[285]

You'll strain your thyroid until you damage it. You may even kill it. I think of a twenty-four-year-old vegan I talked to. Arthritis in her knees, crippling menstrual pain, and a daily dose of Synthroid. "Do you really think your body was meant to fall apart at age twenty-four?" I urged. My information unmoored her but she was desperate. I know exactly how she felt. But her boyfriend was a vegan; so were most of her friends. I don't know where she landed in the end.

You may destroy your stomach like I did. Your hair will dry out, thin, and your skin may get so dry it hurts. Your immune system, built from protein, won't be strong enough to protect you. And it may kick into overdrive from all the plant lectins and their molecular mimicry. Remember who gets autoimmune diseases and who doesn't.

You'll be cold. Then you'll be freezing. You'll be tired and you won't know why. Everything will become such an effort. You won't understand how other people have the energy to go to school and then to work and then out dancing. It's not normal to be that tired. I'm telling you: it's not normal.

And then there's the B12. The terrible sticking point. Just accept it: there are no non-animal sources of B12 and you can end up blind or brain-damaged without it.[286] B12 deficiency also leads to infertility, miscarriage, and maybe Alzheimer's.[287] Just take the damn supplements.

Here's what you'll do to your kids: neurological damage that could well be permanent. Breast-fed infants of vegan mothers can have brain abnormalities from lack of B12.[288] Kids on vegan diets "demonstrated neurological impairments that persisted, even when animal products were added later." Similarly, B12 levels in the blood of formerly vegan children remained low even *after* animal products were added back into their diets. And vegan children scored "substantially lower on tests measuring spatial ability, short-term memory and 'fluid intelligence,' defined as 'the capacity to solve complex problems, abstract thinking ability and the ability to learn.'"[289] Another study found "major skin and muscle wasting ... in 30% of the macrobiotic infants."[290]

One researcher put it bluntly: "There have been sufficient studies clearly showing that when women avoid all animal foods, their babies are born small, they grow very slowly and they are developmentally retarded, possibly permanently.... There's absolutely no question that it's unethical for parents to bring up their children as strict vegans."[291]

In one small community of vegans, twenty-five infants had protein and frank calorie deficiencies, anemia from a lack of both iron and B12, rickets, zinc deficiencies, and retarded growth. One baby died, weighing at five months less than when she was born.[292] I know what I did to myself being a vegan; I shudder when I think of what I could have done to a child.

Soy will make all of the above worse.

You can do a lot of this damage on the standard American diet just as easily. The PUFAs, the sugars, the omega-6s, the plant lectins: it's all there, and all deadly, in the grains and their oils that we were never meant to eat. But you can fix it as a carnivore. You can't as a vegetarian.

And then there's your brain: the depression, the anxiety. Some proportion of you, especially the teenage girls, will end up with full-blown anorexia from trying to be vegetarian. PETA puts their ads with fluffy chicks and baby pigs in magazines aimed at teen girls.

Never mind their endless misogynist ads, the live naked supermod-els in cages: I can't forgive them for going after the teenage girls. One study found that only 17 percent of vegetarian girls consumed enough protein.[293] It's only a matter of time until the tryptophan-deprived brain becomes a disease, then a demon. In another study of teenagers, "All vegetarians weighed themselves more often and were more likely to say that they were dissatisfied with their bodies than nonvegetarians."[294] So it begins. PETA is willing to sacrifice these girls for the cause. I'm not.

You will not live longer. I remember absorbing the "fact" that vegetarians lived longer. Two years, five years, seven years? I didn't know the details but I repeated it to anyone who asked. And of course it's not true. What is true is that people who choose vegetari-anism are a health-conscious group: they also don't smoke or drink and they exercise. Those are the variables that create a longer life span. Compared to the average US American, Seventh-Day Ad-ventists have lower rates of "hypertension, diabetes, arthritis, colon cancer, prostate cancer, fatal CHD in males, and death from all causes."[295] Because Seventh-Day Adventists are supposed to refrain from meat, politicized vegetarians have raised these numbers as a battle cry. But comparing Seventh-Day Adventists to the average US American is absurd, because they are also forbidden to drink alcohol and coffee and they aren't allowed to smoke. They eat substantially more fresh food and substantially fewer doughnuts. Of course they're healthier. If you want to claim that their health is a function of their vegetarian diets, you need to find a cohort to compare them to: a group of people whose diet and lifestyle match that of the Seventh-Day Adventists *except for meat*. Guess what? Those people exist. They're called Mormons. Mormons also abstain from alcohol, coffee, smoking, and lots of the generalized junk of SAD. But they eat meat. Guess who lives longer? Surely you've guessed the punchline: Mor-mons.[296]

But even putting aside all the lifestyle differences that many vegetarians embrace—the abstention from cigarettes and alcohol, the exercising—the all-cause death rate for vegetarian men (0.93%) is *still* a little higher than for omnivorous men (0.89%). For vegetarian women, it's substantially higher (0.86%) than for omnivorous women (0.54%).[297] As early as 1970, vegan women were shown to have higher death rates from heart disease than nonvegan women.[298] And vegetarians are 2.5 times as likely to die from mental and neurological diseases.[299] Nobody told me that.

I'm telling you.

And I'm telling you again that people on low-fat diets are twice as likely to die from violent death or suicide. Death is forever. So is suicide, especially for the people who find the body. My friendship circle lived through a spectacular suicide, and yes, she was an abuse survivor, but weren't we all? She was also a vegan. Her mood disintegrated from depression and fits of anger to paranoid rages until she killed herself. Do I know for a fact that she would have found a way through if she'd eaten some real food? No. The distance between endurance and despair can be measured in so many variables. But I know for myself that a little serotonin can go an awfully long way.

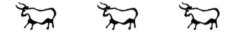

I know what you want to be true, vegetarians. You want to open the circle of concern to everything sentient. With all your hearts, you want us humans to be meant for cellulose or seeds or berries or anything that you believe can't feel pain. And I'm telling you the truth: it doesn't work. What you are made of—bones, blood, brain, heart—needs animals. This is not the universe you wanted. But it's the way the world, always alive and always hungry, works. You can try to live on those other things—the cellulose you can't digest, the seeds that fight back, the berries and their sugar. If you're like me, you'll do it until you're half dead. If you're smarter than me, you'll learn. You want to open that circle, but in fact there's no way out of it. We're all of us, seeded and feathered, rooted and furred, already in it.

Somewhere inside you is an animal that wants to eat. There's no dishonor in that animal. She's the same animal who wants to curl up around her sleeping beloveds, to keep them safe and warm. She's the same animal who comes alive at the smell of rain. She's an animal who belongs here.

She's four million years old. She's in the shape of your teeth, the empty bowl of your one stomach. She's in your stalwart heart, a hundred years strong, surrounded by animal fat. She's in the folds of your brain, and the messages they can carry. Across four million years, those folds grew exquisite, until the messages needed an answer. Your animal found language, art. She answered. She drew what mattered. Go look. The pictures are still there. She left them for you: take, eat, this is the body we have made, predator and prey together. This is the pact, the prayer, our true first communion, not wine, but blood: we are all part of each other.

Bow your head and take aim. Then take your turn.

CHAPTER 5
To Save the World

Start with a sixteen-year-old girl. She has a conscience, a brain, and two eyes. Her planet is being drawn and quartered, species by species. She knows it even while the adults around her play shell games with carbon trade schemes and ethanol. She's also found information that leaves her sickened in her soul, the torment of animals that merges sadism with economic rationality to become the US food supply. Their suffering is both detailed and institutionally distant, and both of those descriptors hold their own horrors. A friend of mine talks about "the thing that breaks and is never repaired." Anyone who has faced the truth about willful or socially-sanctioned cruelty knows that experience: in slavery, historic and contemporary; in the endless sexual sadism of rape, battering, pornography; in the Holocaust and other genocides. You're never the same after some knowledge gets through with you. But our sixteen-year-old has courage and commitment, and now she wants to do what's right.

The vegetarians have a complete plan for her. It's simple. You can create justice for animals, for impoverished humans, and for the earth if you eat grains and beans. That simplicity is part of its appeal, partly because humans have a tendency to like easy rules. But it also speaks to our desire for beauty, that with one act so much that's wrong can be set right: our health, our compassion, our planet.

The problem is they're wrong, not in their attempts to save the world, but in their solution. The moral valuing of justice over power, care over cruelty and biophilia over anthropocentrism is a shift in values that must occur if we are to save this planet. I didn't call this book *The Vegetarian Lie.* I called it *The Vegetarian Myth* for a reason. It's not a lie that animals are sentient beings currently being tortured for our food. It's not a lie that the rich nations are siphoning off the life of the planet for literally oceans full of endless, empty plastic junk. It's not a lie that most people refuse to face the systems of domination—their brute scale—that are destroying us and the earth.

But the vegetarians' solution is a myth based on ignorance, an ignorance as encompassing as any of those dominating systems. Civilization, the life of cities, has broken our identification with the living land and broken the land itself. "The plow is the ... the world's most feared wrecking ball," writes Steven Stoll.[1] For ten thousand years, the six centers of civilization have waged war against our only home, waged it mostly with axes and plows. Those are weapons, not tools. Never mind reparations or repair: no peace is possible until we lay them down.

Those six centers were each driven by a tight cohort of creatures, at the center of which stand an annual plant or two. And humans have been so useful to corn and rice and potatoes, clever enough to conquer perennial polycultures as vast as forests, as tough as prairies, but not smart enough to see we've been destroying the world. The cohort has often included infectious diseases, diseases like smallpox and measles that jumped the species barrier from domesticated animals to humans. Humans who stood in the way of civilization's hunger have been eradicated by the millions through civilization's microbes, the first clear-cut preparing the way for the plow.

This is the ignorance where the vegetarian myth dead ends. Life must kill and we are all made possible by the dead body of another. It's not killing that's domination: it's agriculture. The foods the vegetarians say will save us are the foods that destroy the world. The vegetarian attempt to remove humans from a paradigmatical pinnacle is commendable. And it's crucial. We will never take our true place, one sibling amongst millions, sharing a common journey from carbon to consciousness, sacred and hungry, then back to carbon, without firmly and forever rejecting human dominion.

But in order to save the world we must know it, and the vegetarians don't, not any more than the rest of the civilized, especially the industrially so. Hens driven insane in battery cages are visible to vegetarians; both morally and politically that insistent sight is needed. What are invisible are all the other animals that agriculture has driven extinct. Entire continents have been skinned alive, yet that act goes unnoticed to vegetarians, despite the scale. How do they *not* see it? The answer is they don't know to look for it. We are all so used to a devastated landscape, covered in asphalt and the same small handful of suburban plants, a biotic coup of its own. The whole east coast should be one slow sigh of wetland, interspersed with marsh meadows and old growth forest. It's all gone, replaced by a McMonocrop of houses, shackles of asphalt, the brutal weight of cities.

Where the water goes shy, the trees should thin to savanna and prairie, although even there the wetlands should cradle the rivers. But there's nothing left. The deltas and swamps, bison and black terns, have been turned into soy and wheat and corn. The capitalists say we should turn those into animal units; the vegetarians say we should dump them near the starving; I say we should stop growing them and let the world come back to life. Then we can take our place again, that place that the vegetarians claim to want, our place as participants.

We can dominate or we can participate but there is no way out. That's what no one is telling that sixteen-year-old. The earth is literally dying for wetlands and forests, rivers and prairies. And if humans would simply step aside, the world would do the work of repairing itself. But that repair involves death. It means letting the beavers eat the trees, letting the wolves eat the beavers, letting the soil eat us all. It means taking down every last dam and letting the salmon come home to lay their eggs and be eaten, and in the eating become the forest. This is the world as it should be, resiliently nourishing itself, the gift both given and received. No one is going to tell that sixteen-year-old girl the truth, because there's no one left in her world who knows it.

Letting the beavers come back will mean that wetlands may well cover one-third of the land in places. Those wetlands can't coexist with our roads and suburbs and agriculture. So where does your loyalty lie? Ask yourself that question as if you really mean it. Those wetlands would also feed us forever. To bring the wolves back would require a similar and massive contracture of human activity: they need land, wild land, sturdy with functioning forests and grasslands, not broken by cars, gouged into subdivisions, and coerced into mono-crops. You can't have it both ways, vegetarians. If you want to save this world, including its animals, you can't keep destroying it. And your food destroys it.

If you want rules about what to eat, I can give you some principles. They're slightly more complicated than "Meat Is Murder," but then the living world is complex, and beholding it should leave us all aching with awe. So start with topsoil, the beginning place. Remember, one million creatures per tablespoon. It's alive, and it will protect itself if we stop assaulting it. It protects itself with perennial polycultures, with lots and lots of plants intertwining their roots, adding carbonaceous leaves, and working together with mycelium, bacteria, protozoa, making a new organism between them, the mycorrhiza that talks and nourishes and directs.[2]

Defend the soil with your life, reader: there is no other organism that can touch the intelligence of what goes on beneath your feet.

So here are the questions you should ask, a new form of grace to say over your food. Does this food build or destroy topsoil? Does it use only ambient sun and rainfall, or does it require fossil soil, fossil fuel, fossil water, and drained wetlands, damaged rivers? Could you walk to where it grows, or does it come to you on a path slick with petroleum?

Everything falls into place with those three questions. Those annual monocrops lose on all three counts, unless you live in Nebraska, where it "only" fails the first two. Animal rights philosopher Peter Singer argues that you should only eat animal products if you can see their origin with your own eyes. While I agree with the impulse—to end the denial and ignorance that protect factory farming—this demand has to be much bigger: you should know where every bite of your food comes from. We need to end the denial and ignorance that protect agriculture. The worldview that gives any and all plant foods an automatic pass is profoundly blind to how those very foods devour living communities. Go look at Nebraska, where the native prairie is 98 percent gone. Even if you've never seen an Audubon bighorn or a swift fox, you must surely miss them.

We've all built this living world of gift and need, birth and return. To repair this planet, we must take our sustenance as part of those relationships instead of destroying them. We can pull the forest down or we can eat the deer that live there. We can rip up the grass or we can eat the bison that should stretch across the plains. We can dam the rivers or we can eat the fish that could feed us forever. We can turn biologic processes into commodities until the soil is salt and dust, or we can take our place as another hungering member of an ancient tribe, the tribe of carbon. All flesh is grass, wrote someone named Isaiah in a book I don't usually quote. In Hebrew, the word translated as "flesh" is *basar*, meaning meat, something one eats. Isaiah understood what is no longer physically visible to us, living at the end of the world: we are all a part of one another, made from grass, become meat.

"But food requires destruction," a vegan argued with me, in an e-mail exchange that went exactly nowhere. That is the final myth you must face, vegetarians. Because the food I am proposing, the food of our ancestors, whose paleolithic hearts and souls we still inhabit, does not require destruction. At this moment it would in fact require repair and restitution: the forests and grasslands mended, conquered territory ceded back to the earth for her wetlands. Steven Stoll sums up agriculture: "Humans became parasites of the soil."[3] It's your food that has brought us to the end of the world.

My food builds topsoil. I've watched it happen. The mixture of grasses and trees, cousins in their own right, provides for the animals, who in their turn maintain and nourish by their simple biological functions of eating and excreting. On Joel Salatin's Polyface Farm—the mecca of sustainable food production—organic matter has increased from 1.5 percent in 1961 to 8 percent today. The average right now in the US is 2-3 percent. In case you don't understand, let me explain. A 6.5 percent increase in organic matter isn't a fact for ink and paper: it's a song for the angels to sing. Remember that pine forest that built one-sixteenth of an inch of soil in fifty years? Cue those angels again: Salatin's rotating mixture of animals on pasture is building *one inch of soil annually*.[4]

Peter Bane did some calculations. He estimates that there are a hundred million agricultural acres in the US similar enough to the Salatins' to count: "about 2/3 of the area east of the Dakotas, roughly from Omaha and Topeka east to the Atlantic and south to the Gulf of Mexico."[5] Right now, that land is mostly planted to corn and soy. But returned to permanent cover, it would sequester 2.2 billion tons of carbon every year. Bane writes:

> That's equal to present gross US atmospheric releases, not counting the net reduction from the carbon sinks of existing forests and soils ... Without expanding farm acreage or remov-ing any existing forests, and even before undertaking changes in consumer lifestyle, reduction in traffic, and increases in industrial and transport fuel efficiencies, which are absolutely imperative, the US could become a net carbon sink by chang-ing cultivating practices and marketing on a million farms. In fact, we could create 5 million new jobs in farming if the land were used as efficiently as the Salatins use theirs.[6]

Understand: agriculture was the beginning of global warm-ing. Ten thousand years of destroying the carbon sinks of perennial polycultures has added almost as much carbon to the atmosphere as industrialization (see Figure 5, opposite), an indictment that you, vegetarians, need to answer. No one has told you this before, but that is what your food—those oh so eco-peaceful grains and beans—has done.[7] Remember the ghost acres and the ghost slaves? What you're eating in those grains and beans is ghost meat, down to the bare bones of whole species. There is no reconciling civilization and its foods with the needs of our living planet.

To save the world, we must first stop destroying it. Cast your eyes down when you pray, not in fear of some god above, but in

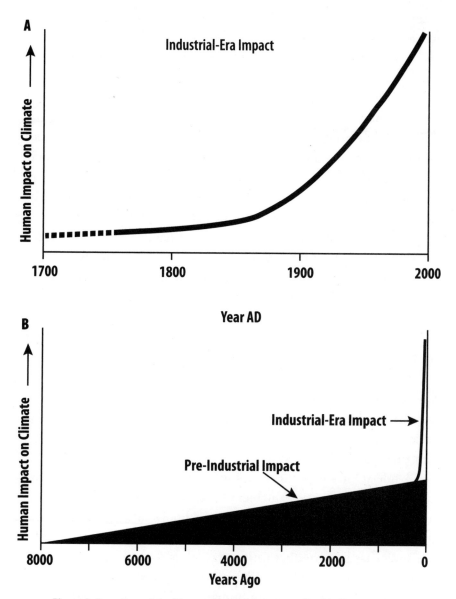

Figure 5. Two views of the history of human impacts on Earth's climate and environment. A: Major impacts began during the industrial era (the last 200 years). B: The changes of the industrial era were preceded by a much longer interval of slower, but comparably important, impacts.

Redrawn from William Ruddiman, *Ploughs, Plagues and Petroleum.*

recognition: our only hope is in the soil, and in the trees, grasses, and wetlands that are its children and its protectors both.

"And why are we not doing this now?" is the clarion call Bane ends with. For a lot of reasons, most of them having to do with power. But a new populism could spring from this need, a serious political movement combining environmentalists, farm activists, animal rights groups, feminists, indigenous people, anti-globalization and relocalization efforts—all of us who are desperate for a new, and living, world.

That's the real reason I've written this book. The earth, our only home, needs that movement, and she needs it now. The only just economy is a local economy; the only sustainable economy is a local economy. Come at it from whichever angle matches your passion, the answers nest around the same central theme: humans have to draw their sustenance from where they live, without destroying that place.

That means that first we must know that place. I can't give you a list of what to eat because I don't know what can live where you do. I can only give you the principles I've already laid out. Then you'll have to ask questions. How much rain falls where you are? What's the terrain, the temperature, the soil? Dairy cattle, for instance, do great things where I live in cold, wet New England. I wouldn't suggest them in dry New Mexico.

Understand my point. Farming—the growing of annual monocrops—will never be sustainable. Our *only* chance is a judicious and humble human participation in perennial polycultures. We can do that poorly, as demonstrated in the overgrazing due to population pressures that is currently turning grasslands to desert the world over. Or we can do it well, like the Fulani of Africa, with a largely unbroken line reaching back to a pre-human time four million years ago.

How much can we change the landscape before participation becomes destruction? Especially when our impact may not be visible for a thousand years? Should we, for instance, use fire? Fire will drive out some species, both plant and animal, and encourage others. Where I live, sugar maples are iconic. Yet five hundred years ago, they wouldn't have been here, or not many of them. The burning practices of Native Americans kept the forest here shifted toward fire-resistant and mast-bearing trees. That information was a shock to my system: don't mess with my maple trees. But Brian Donahue makes the point that as long as there has been a forest in New England, there have been humans living in it.[8] We belong here, too, if we would just behave like it. The pristine forest free of human influence has never existed here, so is it the ideal we should be aiming for?

If so, that ideal must presuppose a devastated landscape somewhere else and an interstate highway system to transport the foods produced out of it. None of this can last: not the devastation, the fossil fuel, the distance. We need to eat where we live and our food must be part of the repair of our home.

Let's look at an example. Do dairy cows belong in New England? In the here and now, as I make my personal and political decisions about breakfast, are cows on the side of good or do they need to be hauled up Mount Doom?

Dairy cattle were brought over from Europe four hundred years ago. Does that rule them out automatically? But if you dig deeper into the past, there were once thirty-three more *genera* of large mammals on this continent, relatives of horses, cows, elephants, giraffes—and not that long ago, a mere 12,000 years. Their absence has left evolutionary widows, trees like honey locust and osage orange that are in decline because they need large herbivores to help them.[9] In that sense, horses and cows were perhaps *reintroduced* with the spread of Europeans. So dig deeper still. Are these new animals similar enough to the ones that are gone, or do their divergences make them destructive assailants on the land base? There were, for instance, once equids here, but they had cloven hooves and no upper teeth. The result of the solid hooves and incisors is "ecological havoc."[10] The feral horses from Europe destroy desert seeps and springs, smother spawning gravel with silt, and strip grasslands to bare dirt. The most in-depth analysis of nineteen study sites found severe damage to "soils, rodents, reptiles, ants, and plants."[11] That damage puts species from desert tortoises to the endangered Lahontan cutthroats at risk.

There are clearly brittle landscapes too fragile for cows—especially for dairy cows—as well. Most of the west is more suited to the animals that were already there—buffalo, pronghorns, elk—and that's what the people there should be eating. So that's a directive: restore the prairie, long grass and short, and the drylands, and return their animal cohorts. Then think long and hard about other megafauna and their place on this continent. Do the grasslands and savannas want them back, or their relatives that still survive? What about the honey locust and osage orange, who need their large seeds to be digested and carried by large herbivores? Is their dying simply evolution at work? If we humans reintroduce some creature that might fulfill that function and restore the range of those trees, is that also evolution? Or is that interference?

And I still need to decide about breakfast.

Cattle on pasture in my climate can easily be sustainable. Joel Salatin is certainly proving that. The model is sound and the climate and rainfall are suitable. But pasture isn't the natural landscape of New England. Forests, wetlands, and marsh meadows are. The Europeans' cows first grazed in those meadows and forests. As the beaver were eradicated, the wetlands and marsh meadows disappeared. Meanwhile, in Europe, experimentation with plant admixtures improved the sustainability of pastures dramatically. How does turning some forest land into pasture compare with the habitat shift of burning? Both of these are activities that, done well, will build topsoil and provide for human sustenance essentially forever. So how much impact are we allowed to have? The entire rainforest is a human project. Small patches are burned by the indigenous like the Lacandon Mayan, and then planted in a succession of eighty different crops, including the vines, shrubs, and trees that will take over when the plot has been abandoned—though "abandoned" is not really an accurate description, as the plot will be revisited in a twenty-year rotation, and will meanwhile produce food, fiber, and building materials, as well as a home for the wild animals that serve as protein.[12]

Which brings me to my point. It wasn't pasture that brought down the northeast forest. It was coal. As long as the human economy was based on wood in this cold climate, people more or less took care of the forest, because they needed it. Coal was what reduced the forest to simply one more commodity, and the land that forests grew on was more profitably used for wool breeds of sheep. What will happen as the price of oil first climbs past what the average household can pay, then past the effort worth retrieving it from the ground? Will New England be cleared from the Atlantic Ocean to the Housatonic River as people freeze to death? Or will the rural areas and private woodlot owners be able to hang onto their parts of this young forest, knowing that without it they, too, will soon freeze? Will we be facing a war not over Middle Eastern oilfields, but over trees in the Berkshires?

And I still need to decide about breakfast.

I can raise these issues, but maybe I can't answer the questions. I know that whatever we're eating has to build soil, and if it doesn't, it has to be struck forever from the human menu. It has to be part of a self-replicating community, where life and death are inseparable in the process of nourishment. Everyone has to give back, through the labor of their life functions, and then through the nutrients stored in their bodies. Our food can't be based on fossil fuel, for nitrogen or energy. Nor can it use fossil water, or indeed any water that empties a river.

Dairy cows, where I live, meet those criteria and more. But is the change in species composition wrought by human-set fire on the acceptable side of the line while the change required for pasture placed in the unacceptable column? Then what we will eat instead will be deer and moose. Both of those, along with bison, migrated here from Eurasia not too long ago, maybe 12,000 years. They filled in niches left empty by the megafaunal extinctions. They're Eurasian transplants, too. Do you see how complicated this gets?

And I still need my breakfast.

In the end, I do have my own answers to offer, of course, but they involve a bit more than drinking soy milk. Agriculture has to stop. It's been a ten thousand year disaster, as life on earth will tell us if we listen. Writes William Catton:

> The breakthrough we called industrialization was fundamentally unlike earlier ones. It did not just take over for human use another portion of the web that had previously supported other forms of life. Instead, it went underground to extract

carrying capacity supplements from a finite and depletable fund ...[13]

As discussed earlier, I think the beginning of the fossil fuel age does mark a new level of human destructiveness, but he's wrong in his characterization of agriculture as simply taking over more ecological niches. Agriculture is extractive: soil is depletable and "peak soil" was ten thousand years ago, on the day before agriculture began. We've been on the down curve ever since.

So agriculture has to stop. It's about to run out anyway—of soil, of water, of ecosystems—but it would go easier on us all if we faced that collectively, and then developed cultural constraints that would stop us from ever doing it again.

Where I live, the wetlands need to return to cover the land in a soft, slow blanket of water. They will be a home for a lush multitude of species, many of which—waterfowl, moose, fish—could feed us. The rivers need to be undammed. And the suburbs and the roads need to be abandoned. I have no great solutions for how to make that economically feasible: I sincerely doubt it's possible. I only know it has to happen, no matter how much we resist. As James Kunstler points out:

> Our suburbs will prove to be a huge liability. They repre-
> sent the greatest misallocation of resources in the history of
> the world. The project of suburbia represents a set of tragic
> choices because it is a living arrangement with no future....
> Our suburbs entail a powerful psychology of previous invest-
> ment that will prevent us from even thinking about reform-
> ing them or letting go of them. There will be a great battle to
> preserve the supposed entitlements to suburbia and it will be
> an epochal act of futility, a huge waste of effort and resources
> that might have been much better spent in finding new ways
> to carry on.[14]

He paints a post-industrial still-life of the suburbs become unliv-able, as oil prices rise and the built environment arranged entirely for cars stops working entirely. Housing is the largest investment the average person has. It will soon be worthless if it's in the suburbs. Most of the world has invested in infrastructure built on a promise of infinite fossil fuel; most of the human race has also reproduced on the premise of infinite food from that same fossil fuel. "Yet nature does not negotiate," writes Richard Heinberg. "The earth is a bounded sphere, and human population growth *will be* reined in."[15]

The house where I sit writing this will not exist in a hundred years. Nothing in me mourns that fact. If all the methane is released from the melted permafrost and the planet is hotter than Venus, there won't even be bacteria left: yes, we *can* kill this planet. *That* is the raging current of grief we all must negotiate if we're to rise to the occasion of this emergency called civilization. In the gentler scenarios, industrial-agricultural society has collapsed, human activity has contracted, and hopefully we have learned a lesson that will be permanently inscribed on every culture to follow. In that case, the wetlands are back, a slow berceuse of species. What's left of this house is perhaps some cinderblocks, the rest of the wood and sheetrock and carpet having melted down between water and time. The road is mostly underwater as well, the asphalt slowly pried apart by the fierce contractions of soil giving birth to ice and the small, persistent hunger of roots. Almost all the houses along this stretch of road have followed the same fate, for the same reasons: they were built on ground stolen from the wetlands, in locations too far from nodes of human activity to be habitable after the final silence of the internal combustion engine.

And the people that live here now? There are far too many of us, many more than the planet can support even using drawdown methods of agriculture and the Haber-Bosch process, the ghost acres from the flayed prairies and emptied oceans. Loren Cordain points to our "absolute dependence" on agriculture, calling it "a path of no return."[16] As many as 80 percent of the calories consumed by humans right now are provided by those annual monocrops. This was set in motion ten thousand years ago when the opioids of annual grass seeds clicked into the pleasure centers of the human brain, and ever since we have been invincible as a cohort, or so we've convinced ourselves. Our very creation myth tells us to dominate, to conquer, to go forth and multiply. No hunter-gatherer is told by god to willfully overshoot the land's carrying capacity, and no marginally rational person would listen to such a god. Cancer, like insanity, spreads with civilization, as I've already quoted. Did Stanislaus Tanchou understand the depth of truth in that sentence? We have become both cancerous and insane as a culture.

Catton compares industrial civilization to the cargo cults of Melanesia. These people had no way to understand how manufactured goods came into existence, and a whole range of religious practices sprang up almost overnight to try to propitiate the spirits to bring more. Are we even fractionally more rational? "The modern Cargoist who expects to be bailed out of this year's ecological predicament by next year's technological breakthrough holds similar beliefs because of his inadequate knowledge of ecology and of technology's role in it. But Cargoist faiths rest upon the quicksand of fundamental ignorance lubricated by superficial knowledge," writes William Catton. [17] Richard Heinberg describes the mass psychology of industrial culture as quasi-religious. "Their pathetic faith in technology turned out to be almost religious in character, as though their gadgets were votive objects connecting them with an invisible but omnipotent god capable of overturning the laws of thermodynamics."[18] Energy cannot be created or destroyed. It really is that simple. We can only hunt, gather, and harvest it. We've taken the energy that was stored—the wood, coal, oil, and gas—and used it to extract nonreplicable resources, like soil and metal, in the service of expanding our species and at the cost of most others. Drawdown and sustainability are not difficult concepts. It's clearly not the arithmetic that's the problem. It's the psychology, which, with equally simple addition, is one part ignorance, one part entitlement, and one part denial. But as Heinberg points out:

> There is an essential lesson here. If we want peace, democracy, and human rights, we must work to create the ecological conditions essential for those things to exist: i.e., a stable human population at—or less than—the environment's long-term

carrying capacity.... The longer we wait, the fewer our options. Social liberals and progressives who fail to talk openly about population and resources issues and to propose workable solutions are merely helping to create their own worst nightmare.[19]

We could ease into energy descent while holding on ferociously to justice, compassion, and the concept of universal human rights. We could. But I see no evidence that we—global or local we—are preparing for that. Instead, industrial civilizations are going to clutch entitlement with one hand and denial with the other. Prove me wrong. Please, show me the evidence, because I am not looking forward to the next fifty years. Without an unassailable commitment to justice and democracy, the contraction of both population and consumption promises to be heartless as well as relentless.

And I still haven't decided about breakfast.

What we are up against is the whole culture. We will not get from here—a planet being sundered before our eyes—to anywhere but hell without a complete revisioning of our way of life. Those of us in rich nations have to accept that we can't do whatever we want, we can't have whatever we want, we can't take whatever we want. Not anymore. The planet has limits: ultimately only so much sunlight falls each day, and only so much of any biotic community can go to feed our species without damage to its integrity. There is an absolute limit, and that boundary has to be respected.

But to state the obvious, this is not a culture that respects boundaries. Agriculture destroys the boundaries of living communities like rivers, prairies, forests, soil. Genetic engineering defies the boundaries of species. Globalization is a contemptuous disregard for the boundaries of local cultures and economies. And rape violates the boundaries of women.

Riane Eisler names this the "dominator model."[20] The idea is that there's a psychological and cultural template that entitles one category of beings to dominate others. Once that's in place, emotionally, intellectually, morally, it can extend itself until it encapsulates the whole culture and every relationship in it.

It's a useless chicken-and-egg project to try to figure out which came first, patriarchy or agriculture, male domination or human domination, because there are examples of each without the other. There are hunter-gatherers who are profoundly patriarchal. There are agriculturalists who are rape-free. It's also useless because it doesn't matter. In the here and now, the system that we live under is a seamless excuse for hierarchy. The core of that dominator model needs to be confronted and dismantled.

I say that core is masculinity. I'm not talking about biological maleness. I mean a psychology based on entitlement, emotional numbness, and a dichotomy of self and other. Masculinity is required in any militarized culture, because those are the psychological traits necessary in soldiers. One can only kill on command if the human impulse to care for one another has been subdued or eradicated. The constant need to turn others into Others is one result: the rejected, "soft" parts of the self are projected outward so they can be destroyed.[21] This is a project that will likely never end as humans do have hearts and souls, and those can never be excised, try as men might. The Viet Nam vets who suffered the worst post-traumatic stress weren't the ones who survived atrocities, but those who committed atrocities.[22]

Masculinity requires what psychologists call a negative reference group, which is a group of people "that an individual ... uses as a standard representing opinions, attitudes, or behaviour patterns to avoid."[23] Boys in patriarchal cultures create negative reference groups as a matter of course. Girls, being socialized to nurture, not dominate, don't.[24] Because the feminine is denigrated in patriarchy, boys' first despised Other is, of course, girls. But once the psychological process is in place, the category "female" can easily be filled in by any group that a hierarchical society needs dominated or eradicated.

A personality with an endless drive to prove itself against another, any other, combined with the entitlement that power brings creates a violation imperative. This means that men in patriarchy feel masculine, like "real men," only when they break boundaries. But being a "real man" is a state that can never be firmly achieved. Writes Robert Jensen:

Be a man.

It is a simple imperative, repeated over and over to men, starting when we are small boys. The phrase is usually connected to one man's demands that another man be "stronger," which is traditionally understood as the ability to suppress emotional reactions and channel that energy into controlling situations and establishing dominance.... When we become men—when we accept the idea that there is something called masculinity to which we should conform—we exchange those aspects of ourselves that make life worth living for an endless struggle for power that, in the end, is illusory and destructive not only to ourselves but to others.[25]

That endless struggle for power results in men committing brutal and violating acts as a matter of course. Psychological profiles of rapists have found "that they are 'ordinary' and 'normal' men who sexually assault women in order to assert power and control over them."[26] We need to be questioning ordinary, normal men and masculinity. Battering is the most common violent crime in the US, committed once every fifteen seconds. It's one of the leading causes of injury and death to women in the US.[27] A Canadian survey found that four out of five female undergraduates had been victims of violence in a dating relationship.[28] The World Health Organization estimates that "one in four women will be raped, beaten, coerced into sex or otherwise abused in her lifetime, sometimes with fatal consequences."[29] Anything happening on this scale is clearly normal, a part of everyday life, the behavior into which a global culture of male dominance is socializing men as a matter of course.

The real brilliance of patriarchy is that it sexualizes acts of oppression. For the perpetrators, violation and brutality lead to arousal. In any other circumstance, the same acts would be recognized as hateful. Witness Abu Ghraib. When men are stripped, put in postures of submission, and then photographed, the power is obvious, the oppression clear, and the world is outraged. Meanwhile, women and girls are bought, sold, raped, and displayed as a matter of course, and the world can't get enough. There are entire countries balancing their budgets on sex trafficking.[30]

We will never dismantle misogyny as long as domination is eroticized. But we will also never stop racism, and that insight is one that the Left is refusing to grapple with.[31] Nor will we mount an effective resistance to fascism, since, as Sheila Jeffereys points out, fascism's root is ultimately the eroticization of domination and subordination.[32] Fascism is essentially a cult of masculinity.

It's possible to have a culture that lives within its landbase without respecting human rights, as discussed earlier. But I believe that the dominant culture will never untangle misogyny, racism, and militarism from anthropocentrism, even if that were a morally defensible project. Alongside agriculture, this culture also has to abandon the project of masculinity. As Derrick Jensen says:

> Another way to talk about people not caring what happens to the world is to talk about rape and child abuse. ... [Perpetrators] include respected members of this society. Within this culture, they're normal people. Their behavior has been normalized. If normal people within this culture are raping and beating even those they purport to love, what chance is there that they will not destroy the salmon, the forests, the oceans, the earth?[33]

We have a whole lot of bad habits to give up, and our sentimental attachments are not the answer. For instance, the leading religions of the planet are all variations on the theme of domination, and they've had a few thousand years to prove that yes, they really mean it. The planet is in shreds; the indigenous displaced; slavery a way of life only temporarily veiled by distance and fossil fuel; male supremacy is saturated with sexual sadism; all of it a dictate from the big boy himself. Gore Vidal calls monotheism "the greatest disaster ever to befall the human race."[34] And, yes, people have created beauty from these religions. They've even fashioned calls for justice. But at least admit that both beauty and justice have been a net loss under their reign.

We can do better. We have to. Most of us are living in a culture long since broken from our native animism. But we could rationally choose a spiritual base on which to build the culture we need. Writes Stephen Harrod Buhner:

> The most "primitive" peoples, living deeply embedded in their "environment," all practice ceremonies and rituals that affirm and nourish the interconnectedness, the interbeing of the human tribe with the rest of the Earth family. This would indicate that the propensity to lose this connection is not just a modern phenomenon but is rooted deep within our humanity. We moderns, however, in our arrogance and "enlightenment," have ridiculed such practices, attempted to assign them to the realm of superstition. Ritual has become "empty ritual." Thus our connections are in tatters and the world torn asunder. Having ridiculed such rituals, we did not participate in them; not participating in them, we lost our place in the world. And now, how are we to recover our ecological self? Mere ecological ideas, no matter how deep, cannot save us.[35]

An animist ethic must arise from both our intellectual passion for a life-affirming culture and from the direct experience of our spiritual connection to all beings. Our spiritual practices, whether ancient or new, must provide for recognition of the sentience of those beings and an attitude of abiding humility and awe for our living planet. Perhaps there are beliefs and practices of our varied cultures that can be brought along, anything to do with political resistance, compassion, justice, resilience, tolerance. But the core of dominator religions will always remain authoritarian, fundamentalist, hierarchical, and biocidal. It's my conclusion that these religions need to be abandoned. It's up to those of you who think otherwise to prove me wrong.

And we're still a long way from breakfast.

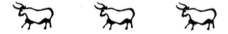

One reason I hesitate to suggest specific foods as morally and ecologically good is that personal food decisions are ultimately a lifestyle choice. And these kinds of personal choices, particularly when they involve buying something, have been embraced by the mainstream environmental movement as solutions. They aren't. If you hear nothing else in this book, hear this: there is no personal solution. And this reifying of individual action cuts right to the heart of the divergence between liberals and radicals.

So here's the basic education in revolution that you didn't get in public school. There are two cardinal differences between liberalism and radicalism. The first can be characterized as idealism versus materialism. Liberalism is idealist. The crucible of social reality is the realm of ideas, in concepts, language, attitudes. In contrast, radicalism is materialist. Radicals see society as composed of actual institutions—economic, political, cultural—which wield power, including the power to use violence.

The second disagreement is on the primary social unit. Liberalism is individualist, locating the basic organization of society in the individual. Hence, liberal strategies for political change are almost exclusively individual actions. For radicals, the basic social unit is a class or group, whether that's racial class, sex caste, economic class, or other grouping. Radicalism of whatever stripe understands oppression as group-based harm. For liberals, defining people as members of a group *is* the harm. In contrast, radicals believe that identifying your interests with others who are dispossessed—and developing loyalty to your people—is the first, crucial step in building a liberation movement.

Liberals essentially think that oppression is a mistake, a misunderstanding, and changing people's minds is the way to change the world. Hence, liberals place a tremendous emphasis on education as a political strategy. Radicals understand oppression as a set of interlocking institutions, and, one way or another, the strategy for liberation involves direct confrontation with power to take those institutions apart.

The Left in this country has embraced liberalism to the point of becoming completely unhitched from any notion of actually being effective. Activism has turned into one big group therapy session. It doesn't matter what we accomplish—what matters is how we *feel* about it. The goal of any action isn't to change the material balance of power, it's to feel "empowered" or to feel "community" or to feel our hearts open to our inner children because our mean, mean mothers never loved us, and all of it is endless and self-referential and useless. And the people who get caught up in this workshop culture will insist that their precious little navels have something to do with changing the world. Meanwhile, the planet is being eviscerated. If you want to do this with your life, well, it's your life, but please don't pretend that you're changing the world.

The related dead end of individualism is the extreme personal purity of the "lifestyle activists." Understand: the task of an activist is not to negotiate systems of power with as much personal integrity as possible—it's to dismantle those systems. Neither of these approaches—personal psychological change or personal lifestyle choices—is going to disrupt the global arrangements of power. They're both ultimately liberal approaches to injustice, rerouting the goal from political change to personal change. This is easier, much easier, because it makes no demands on us. It requires no courage or sacrifice, no persistence or honor, which is what direct confrontations with power must require. But personal purity only asks for shopping and smugness. The mainstream version involves hybrid cars, soy milk, soy burgers, and soy babies, and checking off the "green power" option on your electric bill. On the very fringe, there is a more extreme version which offers a semi-nomadic life of essentially mooching off the employed. To point out the obvious: power doesn't care. Power doesn't notice the existence of anarchist freegans and it certainly doesn't care if they eat out of dumpsters. Power will only care when you build a strategic movement against it. Individual action will never be effective. To quote Andrea Dworkin, we need organized, political resistance.[36] Rosa Parks on her own ended up in jail. Rosa Parks plus the courage, sacrifice, and political will of the whole Black community of Montgomery, Alabama ended segregation on the public transportation system.

And what about breakfast?

I'm going to assume that you know our planet is in trouble. Maybe you mostly turn from the depths of that knowledge, afraid of its emotional acid. Or maybe you live with it like barbed wire tightening around your heart. The promise of personal solutions can ease both denial and despair: most of us are a mixture of those. So if you need your personal fix, here are the three most effective things you can do.

Refrain from having children. That's far and away the single most powerful lifestyle choice you can make for the planet. Understand there are at least six billion more people than the planet can support, already here. I'm speaking as someone who likes children. I've got a green card in Narnia (and don't worry, I'm a registered voter in the Republic of Heaven). I've had the longing that feels like a physical ache. Never mind my mother's craven lust for grandchildren. Yes, it's sad, but what humans are doing to the planet, the endgame of ten thousand years of human entitlement, is much worse than sad. The children of polar bears are now starving to death on the shrinking ice. The children of amphibians as a genera are about to go extinct. The nonexistent children of the already extinct flowering plants in Szechuan are gone because humans have eradicated their pollinators. That's 130 million years of evolution we've wiped from the planet. We have to measure our personal longings against the damage to our home and we have to let that damage be real to us, emotionally, intellectually, spiritually. It's hard to do this when our immediate needs are being met: the lights are on, the cupboards full. Still, that is our adult knowledge now, and our final adult task.

Number two is to stop driving a car. You'll quickly discover the structural impediments to car-free living. The entire built environment has been rearranged for the demands of the automobile, demands that are completely at odds with the needs of human community. US Americans use much more fossil fuel than Europeans, not just because we're fixated on our individual entitlements, but because we were foolish enough to let suburbs, with their segregated distances between home, work, and material goods like food, become our dominant living pattern. This pattern, with all its immense investment in infrastructure, will collapse as the oil age dribbles to a close. New Orleans is going to look like a baby shower in comparison.

Number three is to grow your own food. The two thousand miles that your average bite travels has to shrink to walking distance before the oil runs out and the temperature rises any higher. Your backyard is as good as it gets. When you're hungry enough, your dogs and cats will be replaced by pigs and chickens, and your sterile monocrop of lawn will become a polyphonous and intimate tumble of food. You'll learn what I did about nitrogen and soil, animals and plants, or eventually be left with dead dust. Teach yourself, your friends, your neighbors: a few of them are nervous. The rest will join soon enough.

Perhaps we're getting closer to breakfast?

We are getting closer to some truths that must be faced. One is that despite the deepest longings of your hearts, vegetarians, you are wrong. To save this world we must know it, and then take our place inside it. As long as I believed the annual grains of a plant-based diet would save the world, I couldn't see that they were destroying it. This exact moment—reading these words—will take courage. I know you've got it. Are you willing to use it?

Your ideology is in the way of the adult knowledge this culture needs and the political movement that must spring from it. It's also obstructing the well-being of your own animal body, a body you need to inhabit, not punish. Maybe it helps to know that you haven't been cheating or binging or backsliding: you've been starving. I also know what you'll do next. You'll sign on to a vegan message board or grab John Robbins off the shelf and try to plug the puncture wounds I've made in your identity. Believe me, I know.

And once you're in freefall, after these concepts begin their slow, soaking pressure, or after a few meals of real food and the flood of well-being they release in you, I know what will happen next. You'll have to start telling—confessing—to your friends. And some of them will hate you. Remember this: you can get new friends. You can't get a new body. You also can't get a new planet. Does it help to know this is a cult mentality? Or will that only be a balm afterward, when "recovering vegan" starts to coalesce as a new identity? There are also people who will be relieved. Your mother, for instance. And you know you've grown up when you can tell your mom she was right.

Then there are the political truths. For instance, the nature of civilization, its unsustainability, as well as its destruction of human rights and human culture. Writes Hugh Brody, my argument here pays no attention to class or even to nation. Those who are agriculturalists, humans who live by remodeling the land, are the peoples whose story is some version of Genesis. We live outside any one garden that can meet our needs and growing population ... We are doomed to defend this place against enemies of all kinds: we know that just as we have conquered, others can displace us. This mixture of agriculture and warfare is the system within which farms and towns and nation-states and colonial expansion have an inner and shared coherence. The worldview and daily preoccupations of the peasant farmer and the twenty-first-century executive have much in common. The one is able to dominate, exploit, and thrive far more efficiently than the other. But their intellectual devices, their categories of thought, and their underlying interests may well be the same. They speak one another's language, as it were; for all the inequalities between them, they can do business together.[37]

There's also the hell that we're making for animals, both domestic and wild, the CAFOs and the shrinking ice, the cornfed cows and the oil-sickened birds: *the cause is the same*. It's called civilization, especially its consumptions, including its food. If you're against the one, you have to be against the other.

And finally, liberal remedies will never serve a radical analysis. There is an inherent contradiction in understanding that systems of power must be dismantled while only embracing personal solutions. To put that more bluntly: if agriculture is a war, why aren't we fighting back?

We've almost reached breakfast. Hang in there.

In the broadest strokes, we need a multilayered approach to setting the world right. The first set of tasks revolves around inoculating people against future fascism. Why? Because civic society is going to be under some tremendous strains very soon. As the basic arrangements of industrial society fail, fascism is one likely outcome. Desperate people are vulnerable to easy, authoritarian solutions, especially ones with scapegoats. The first things we're likely to lose are human rights and democracy. Teach people about direct democracy, get local participatory governments in place, and defend the concept of universal human rights at all costs, especially if you work with children. Forget the Pledge of Allegiance. What kids really should be reciting is the United Nations Universal Declaration of Human Rights, and not to a piece of fabric but facing each other. Start a town meeting where you live. In New England, we have a living tradition of local self-government. Vermont still runs by town meeting. Learn how to do it. Even if you can't actually transform the government where you live into a direct democracy right away, get the idea out there and start practicing with whoever will come. These are skills and concepts we are going to need.

Second is building local economies, especially local food networks, and all the survival skills for a post-petroleum world. This is also the place where we need a new culture and new enculturation practices to replace the life patterns to which we've been socialized. Our entire social, spiritual, sexual well-being is scripted around a happy heterosexual nuclear family with two cars, two kids, and enough consumer junk to outfit a third world village. We need a totally different psychological narrative. Some of us have tried to create that, but we're so invisible as to be nonexistent to the culture at large.

And we need new food that protects prairies and forests and wetlands, food that's a partnership between animals and plants, soil and us. We need a spiritual practice that keeps us connected to the sentience of the world, and a sexual practice that begins in justice.

But that new culture can't just be an alternative. It has to be *self-consciously oppositional* to the dominant culture. That means it has to encourage and support organized political resistance. It doesn't mean everyone has to do direct action. There all kinds of reasons—legitimate, rational reasons—for people to refrain, ranging from familial responsibilities to physical disability to spiritual beliefs. But even if we're personally not on the front lines, we have to support the people who are willing and able to do what's necessary. We need a true culture of resistance that actually supports a resistance movement. Because thirdly, we need those direct confrontations with power. In the immortal words of Frederick Douglass, "Power concedes nothing without a demand. It never has and it never will."

In some ways it's very simple: where does it hurt? Where does your body hurt, where does your land hurt? Then ask, who's in charge of inflicting that pain? Then ask, where are they weak, and where are you strong? Enough people could stop global warming, also known as catastrophic climate change. And no, not by buying energy-saving light bulbs, but by standing between fossil fuels and what's left of our planet. Massive civil disobedience is one tactic that could do that. There are also others.[38] Industrial culture is in fact very vulnerable as it's utterly dependent on an infrastructure of oil, gas, electricity, and highways. Yet not one major environmental group is organizing to actually stop the daily biocide: over a hundred species, each and every day. Why? Are we too attached to this way of life? Are we too afraid of the consequences of fighting back? Do we not even know how to think in terms of actually defending our planet? It's so much easier to believe in fairytales, the eco-technotopia of solar panels and hybrid cars. Yet solar panels depend on materials like gallium and indium. Never heard of those? That should be a clue to how rare they are. We've already seriously depleted these substances. And from the mining to the manufacturing, it all depends on an industrial platform that is about to collapse. Meanwhile, biodiesel is a net energy loss. I'm sorry to spoil the story, but there is no techno-fix to get us to happily ever after. Only the end of this long, slow war—its occupations, its atrocities—will.

It's time to put away the fairytales, all of them, and assume our responsibilities, the adult responsibilities that begin with adult knowledge. Our planet needs us. She needs us to think like healers and act like warriors. And if you think that's a contradiction, then get out of the way.

And now, finally, it's time for breakfast.

I'll pause above this food, and know I am of this world, carbon and breath like my parents, my siblings, the creatures great and small, single-celled or green, that create the miracle the rest of us consume. They gave me this body and the air it needs, the food it eats. All they ask is that I take my place, a predator, dependent and beholden, until I am prey. All they ask is that I see: being a part of it, what my body needs is the same as what my land needs. Respect for physical integrity is an absolute; every relationship, each instance of give and take, must begin in mutuality, and end in an awed and tender intimacy. We owe our bodies what we owe the world; we must inhabit both and, in the act of inhabiting, nourish both. This food must also be an apology for what my kind has done, and part of the repair. It must protect this land, and extract from me the promise of more.

My food is those things, all of them. It's based on the forests and grasses that nestle this planet in soil and air. It's mostly the animals themselves I eat, and their offspring, their milk, in the knowledge that I am one such animal, descended from teeth and fur and hunger as well. Some of them—the cows, the pigs—came here recently, like me, from other continents. Some of them—the deer, the moose—came here longer ago. Others—the salmon, the wild turkey—have been here forever. But they all have the lives they were meant to have, and in living those lives, they participate in cycles of water and nutrients, birth and death. They eat what they hunger for; they have what they need; and they help make more, more soil, more species, which is another way of saying: more home, more food. This food repairs the physical world, the ten thousand-year rupturing gash of agriculture.

It also goes some way toward repairing human community. I know the farms and farmers, my neighbors, and I give my money to actual people doing real work—useful, good, honorable work—not fictitious persons created to accumulate wealth without conscience. This food has also repaired my body to the extent that anything can.

I have looked my food in the eye. I have raised some of it myself, loved it when it was small and defenseless. I have learned to kill. And I've learned to say my own grace. It's a prayer of thank you, a petition for the unfolding communion I call home, and a promise to protect the world entire, to stop the agonizing bleed of species and the rising scorch of heat.

To save the world we must know it. We must face where the damage lies—what human activities, in whatever mixture of hubris and ignorance, have done, no matter what it means to our identities, our securities, our dreams.

But to save the world we must also, in the end, save it. So leave everything but your courage and join the battle.

Then join the feast.

Acknowledgements

First, I need to thank some people that I have never met. Foremost among them is the late Dr. Weston A. Price, whose work produced a miracle in my life. I also want to thank the indomitable Sally Fallon Morell for her tireless efforts to educate the public about Price's research. I owe thanks to many other doctors, writers, and activists who are advocates for protective and nourishing foods, especially the late Dr. Robert Atkins, Kaayla Daniel, Drs. Mary Dan and Michael Eades, Dr. Mary Enig, Dr. Malcolm Kendrick, Julia Ross, Dr. Ron Schmid, and Gary Taubes.

I would like to thank my volunteer army of proofreaders, who saved me from untold humiliations: Roxanne Amico, Jorge Chang, Valija Evalds, Rita Franz, Heather Glista, Jen Hartley, Annemarie Monahan, Paul Pigman, Bee Whitner, Patricia Willis, and Jon Zaiglin. A special thank you to my proofreading lieutenants, who made this book both more righteous and more readable: Rhea Becker, Estela López, Paul Seidman, and Rebecca Whisnant. Warm thanks to Dr. Michael Eades for making the book more scientifically accurate and for his support. Theresa Noll, my editor, did wonderful things to help this book fledge. I also want to thank Kathryn Price who gave me a place to live while I finished writing.

I need to thank my friends and colleagues in the feminist anti-pornography movement who give me hope when my courage flags: Gail Dines, Matt Ezzell, Bob Jensen, Rebecca Whisnant, and Patricia Willis.

A huge thank you and a pile of chocolate frogs to Aric McBay for his: beautiful cover and gorgeous layout; endless patience with my computer Luddism; and high humor, strategic brilliance, and basic human decency. I feel very sorry for anyone who doesn't have their own personal Aric.

My parents, Victoria and Egils Evalds, have my gratitude for teaching me that the ease of conformity is not worth the price. The friendship and support of my sister, Valija Evalds, is a continuous trip to Narnia. Susan Gesmer has been a loyal and generous friend for over twenty years. Annemarie Monahan stood by me through the worst of it—surgery, pain clinics, and morphine. She also said yes to chickens.

Finally, a profound thank you to Derrick Jensen, publisher, comrade, and friend. He believed in me and in this book before a single word had been written.

Appendix

Symptoms of Hypoglycemia:

Here's a list of questions developed by the venerable Dr. Robert Atkins to diagnose hypoglycemia.

- Do you have an inexplicable obsession with food?
- A habit of night eating?
- A tendency to binge?
- A craving for such carbohydrate foods as sweets, pastas and breads?
- Do you nibble all day long when food is available?
- A strong desire to eat again shortly after you've eaten to fullness?
- Do you consider yourself a compulsive eater? Have you ever said, "I only wish I could control my eating behavior?"
- Do you have specific symptoms of ill health, such as the ones I'm about to list, that lessen or vanish as soon as you eat? Do you suffer:
- Irritability?
- Inexplicable drops in your strength and stamina at various times throughout the day—often overwhelming bouts of fatigue, especially in the afternoon?

- Mood swings?
- Difficulty in concentrating?
- Sleep difficulties—often a need for considerable quantities of sleep, sometimes a habit of waking from a sound sleep?
- Anxiety, sadness and depression for which there's no situational explanation?
- Dizziness, trembling, palpitations?
- Brain fog and loss of mental acuity?

(From Robert C. Atkins, M. D., *Dr. Atkins' New Diet Revolution* (New York: Avon Books, 1997), p. 39.)

If any of this sounds familiar, you're doing damage every time you eat. You're asking your body to produce and absorb too much insulin, way more than it was built to handle. Listen to your body: you shouldn't be dizzy, trembling, and melting down every few hours. And eventually the damage will be permanent.

Resources

The Weston A. Price Foundation

http://www.westonaprice.org

Founded by Sally Fallon, the foundation aims to educate the public about Price's work and the primacy of traditional animal-source foods to human health. They do political advocacy, like lobbying against the soy industry, and they have a legal arm that defends farmers. Local chapter leaders can help you find pasture-raised meat and raw dairy products. The site contains a veritable orgy of information. Hands down, the best nutrition site on the web.

Also see Sally Fallon and Mary Enig's book, *Nourishing Traditions: The Cookbook that Challenges Politically Correct Nutrition and the Diet Dictocrats.*

Julia Ross

http://www.moodcure.com

Julia Ross runs The Recovery Systems Clinic, where depression, addiction, and eating disorders are treated using a protein-rich diet combined with amino acid supplements. Her book, *The Mood Cure*, is a must for anyone who wants to understand the connection between nutrition and mental illness. I have personally seen her approach work miracles.

Drs. Mary Dan and Michael Eades
http://www.proteinpower.com
The authors of *Protein Power* and *The Protein Power Lifeplan*, among other titles. They provide very accessible explanations of how the human body is meant for animal products, what happens to us when we stray from our evolutionary path, and how to restore our health.

Soy Online Service
http://www.soyonlineservice.co.nz/index.htm
A wealth of information about the dangers and politics of soy.

Eat Wild
http://www.eatwild.com
Jo Robinson's site explains the benefits of pasture-feeding to animals, the earth, and us. She has a state-by-state list of grass-based farms that sell directly to consumers. Also see her book, *Pasture Perfect*.

Local Harvest
http://www.localharvest.org
A great resource for finding local farms and food.

Wise Food Ways
http://www.wisefoodways.com
Jessica Prentice is the woman who brought us the word *locavore*. Her book, *Full Moon Feast: Food and the Hunger for Connection*, is not to be missed, especially if you are a recovering vegetarian.

Eat Local Challenge
http://www.eatlocalchallenge.com
Where the locavores are. Learn about the Eat Local Challenge and find out how other people are doing it.

Beyond Vegetarianism

http://www.beyondveg.com

A good resource for those who need support while questioning their vegetarianism.

The International Network of Cholesterol Skeptics

http://www.thincs.org

A great place to start if you're scared of animal fats. Articles, books, discussion, and news from doctors and scientists defending protective and nourishing foods.

Dr. Malcolm Kendrick

Cholesterol and Heart Disease

http://www.youtube.com/watch?v=i8SSCNaaDcE

Watch Dr. Kendrick demolish the Lipid Hypothesis in one minute, seventeen seconds.

Endnotes

Chapter One

1   Mollison, p. 205.

2   Paulson.

3   Quoted in Manning, *Against the Grain*, p. 24.

4   The US Census Bureau considers farming a statistically insignificant occupation.

5   Prechtel, p. 347-349.

6   Salatin.

7   Lappé, p. 70.

8   See Chapter 3.

Chapter Two

1   The apple's version of a starter home in a decent school district.

2   Åredale.

3   "What is a Fruitarian?"

4   Pollan, *Botany*, p. 55.

5   Åredale.

6   For the non-gardeners, a word of explanation. The fruit trees that you might see in people's backyards are purchased as saplings from nurseries. There are probably a few hobbyists left doing their own grafting at home, but the vast majority of that work is done by professionals.

7   "What is a Fruitarian?"

8   Stout.

9   Mollison.

10 Ibid., p. 205.

11 Ibid., p. 207.

12 Bruhner, p. 165.

13 Mollison, p. 205

14 Buhner, p. 165.

15 Stoll.

16 For you non-gardeners, "bolting" is what lettuce does when the weather gets warm. It sends up a flower stalk almost overnight

and tries to set seed, becoming too bitter to eat in the process. That bitterness is the plant's way of protecting its young, turning away predators by making itself unpalatable.

17 Mollison, p. 192.

18 Ibid., p.192.

19 Phillips, p. 30.

20 Pollan, *Botany*, p. xvi.

21 Ibid.

22 Ibid., p. xxi.

23 Pollan, *Omnivore's Dilemma*, p. 323.

24 Williams, "Wanted: More Hunters."

25 Pollan, *Omnivore's Dilemma*, p. 322.

26 Caufield, p. 53.

27 Rindos.

28 Steckel and Rose, p. 4.

29 Manning, *Against the Grain*, p. 37.

30 Sahlins.

31 Price and Gebauer, p. 191.

32 Pollan, *Botany*, p.117.

33 Buhner, p. 199.

34 Allport, p. 121.

35 Wadley and Martin, p. 96-105.

36 Eades and Eades, *Protein Power LifePlan,* p. 17.

37 And the so-called "Great Plowing" was done before the invention of the internal combustion engine. More than a million acres of prairie were decimated by humans hitched to draft animals.

38 Stoll, p. 30.

39 Paulson.

40 Hillel, p. 50.

41 Ibid., p. 75.

42 Ibid., p. 4.

43 Ibid., p. 4.

44 Ibid., p. 107.

45 Ibid., p. 107.

46 Ibid., p. 103.

47 Manning, *Against the Grain*, p. 40.

48 "Malaria Facts/CDC Malaria."

49 Stoll, p. 14.

50 Hillel, 106.

51 "Prairies of Illinois."

52 "Tallgrass Prairie Project."

53 Tatum.

54 Ferber, p. 24.

55 "Loblolly Marsh Wetland Preserve."

56 Jackson, p 4.

57 Purdy.

58 Mollison, p. 183.

59 Hillel, p. 163.

60 Jackson, p. 113.

61 Ibid., p. 121.

62 Mollison, p. 183.

63 Hillel, p. 82.

64 "Swainson's Warbler."

65 Pearce, p. 24.

66 Ibid., p. 24.

67 Ibid., p. 24.

68 Ibid., p. 30.

69 Ibid., p. 24.

70   Ibid., p. 109.

71   Ibid., p. 110.

72   Ibid., p. 3.

73   Did anyone ever tell you that the Colorado River delta once held beavers and jaguars? Did you even know there was a delta? There won't be for long: the Colorado hasn't reached its delta since 1993. See Pearce, p. 196.

74   Ibid., p. 48.

75   Ibid., p. 83.

76   Ibid., p. 84.

77   Williams, "Last Line," p. 56.

78   Ferber, p. 24.

79   Williams, "Last Line," p. 57.

80   Williams, "America's River," p. 30.

81   "The Struggle to Save Salmon in the Klamath Basin."

82   "Keystone Species."

83   "2002 Fish Die-Off Facts & Articles."

84   Derrick Jensen, p. 696. If you haven't read *Endgame*, put this book down and go get it. Now.

85   Donahue. See especially Chapter 5, "The Town Forest," pp. 217-278.

86   Ibid., p. 249.

87   The status of women is the most potent variable in controlling population growth.

88   I know I'm dating myself here.

89   Brumberg, p. 63.

90   Mercifully, this site has since been taken down. I hope its absence means that Peter is in recovery rather than dead.

91   "Inedia." The rest of the breath-arian quotes are from the same article.

92   Having grown both the heirloom and the Cornish x Rocks, I can personally attest to their astounding growth rate.

93   See Chapter 4.

94   Quoted in Buhner, p. 39.

95   Prentice, p. 215.

96   Vidal, *United States*.

97   See Chapter 3.

98   Merchant.

99   Hochschild, p. 2.

100 "Human facial recognition is a highly specialized ability, and it seems to be pre-wired before birth in specific visual processing areas of the brain.... An infant's inborn ability to recognize a generalized face is apparently evolutionarily quite primitive ... [T]he infant begins with the prototype female "protoface" pre-wired visually into the midbrain, and then later utilizes the cortical areas to add additional visual recognition cues, such as the hairline and ear." See Malmstrom.

101 Scrunton, p. 127.

102 Pollan, *Omnivore's Dilemma*, p. 321.

103 Roosevelt, p. 240.

104 Pollan, *Omnivore's Dilemma*, p. 321.

105 Ibid., p. 322.

106 The captive dolphin's female relatives will try to rescue her.

107 Margulis and Sagan.

108 Derrick Jensen, p. 138. And I meant it about buying this book right now.

109 Did we domesticate them or did they domesticate us? From the bacteria's perspective, we could be the dumb beasts that feed and house them: do we talk on Christmas Eve? See "Bacteria and Human Body Weight."

110 Kemmerer.

111 Lauck, p. 30.

112 Ibid., p. 22.

113 Berry, forward to Lauck, p. xiii.

114 Siegel. Lincoln also stopped other boys from smashing turtles against trees and setting them on fire, two activities among the many that I will never understand. See also Shenk.

115 Buhner, p. 142.

116 Ibid., p. 43.

117 Lauck, p. xvi.

118 Buhner, p.145.

119 Allport, p.108.

120 Buhner, p.190.

121 Ibid., p. 196.

122 Ibid., p. 172.

123 Ibid., p. 162.

124 Ibid., p. 181.

125 Ibid., p. 183.

126 Ibid., p. 183.

127 Ibid., p. 184.

128 Ibid., p. 24.

129 Ibid., p. 145.

130 Ibid., p. 196.

131 Ibid., p. 172.

132 Ibid., p. 175.

133 Ibid., p. 197.

134 Ibid., p. 189.

135 Ibid., p. 37.

136 Ibid., p. 33.

137 Ibid., p. 228.

138 Patzin.

139 Buhner, p. 228.

140 Ibid., p. 228.

141 Ibid., p. 172.

Chapter 3

1 Ekarius, p.65.

2 Mackie.

3 Ekarius, p. 62.

4 Mackie.

5 Thereby rendering the concept of "domestication" rather useless: it's not what humans do, it's what nature does, and it's not an act of power, oppression, or superior intelligence, but how all species act with and upon each others' genomes.

6 Mackie.

7 Ibid.

8 Rodney K. Heitschmidt and Jerry W. Stuth, eds., *Grazing Manage-*

ment: *An Ecological Perspective,* quoted in Carol Ekarius *Small-Scale Livestock Farming,* p. 59.

9   Ekarius, p. 59.

10   Pollan, *Omnivore's Dilemma,* p. 77.

11   Ibid., p. 78.

12   Ibid., p. 78.

13   Ibid., p. 78.

14   Ibid., p. 78.

15   Pyle, p. 94.

16   "The Welfare of Sows in Gestation Crates."

17   Motavalli.

18   Pollan, *Omnivore's Dilemma,* p. 222.

19   Here are my figures. I counted the beef and pork as "lean," since pasture-feeding results in much leaner meat than grain-feeding. The government database (see note 22 below) shows lean beef and pork as 55 calories per once, which is 880 calories per pound.

3,000 eggs x 70 calories each
    = 210,000 calories
1,080 whole chickens x 1,300 calories
    each = 1,404,000 calories
2,000 lbs of beef x 880 calories =
    1,760,000 calories
2,500 lbs of pork x 880 calories =
    2,200,000 calories
50 tom turkeys = 643,300
50 hen turkeys = 482,550
50 rabbits = 100, 200

20   Motavalli.

21   Lozier et al.

22   The traditionally-valued fats and fattier cuts would result in even higher calories and, obviously, more grams of fat, tipping the balance even further toward the superiority of beef. Calorie amounts were taken from two government databases, National Heart, Lung and Blood Institute at http://www.nhlbi.nih.gov/health/public/heart/obesity/lose_wt/fd_exch.htm and USDA Nutrient Data Library at http://riley.nal.usda.gov/NDL.

23   Motavalli.

24   A tiny amount is also liberated by lightning.

25   Pollan, *Omnivore's Dilemma,* p. 43.

26   Ibid., p. 43.

27   Manning, "Oil We Eat," p. 39.

28   Fritz Haber arrived home to a hero's welcome in Berlin. His wife, chemist Clara Immerwahr, reacted rather differently. She shot herself in the heart with his military pistol out in their garden in horror at what he had become. Later on that same morning, Haber road off to oversee further gas attacks. Haber himself was Jewish. He had to flee Germany in 1933. Some of his relatives were killed by Zyklon

B in concentration camps. He himself died alone in a hotel room in Switzerland. His son Hermann committed suicide in 1946. A more complete story of the horrors of racism, patriarchy, militarization, and industrialization would be hard to find.

29 Manning, "Oil We Eat," p. 41.

30 Pyle, p.92.

31 Pollan, *Omnivore's Dilemma*, p. 67.

32 Pyle, p. 107.

33 Ibid.

34 Motavalli.

35 Manning, *Against the Grain*, p.42.

36 Hemenway, p. 6.

37 Pollan, *Omnivore's Dilemma*, p. 46.

38 See Chapter 4.

39 Pyle, p. 91.

40 Ibid., p. 92.

41 Ibid., p. 42.

42 Ibid., p. 25.

43 Ibid., p. 25.

44 Ibid., p. 29.

45 Pollan, *Omnivore's Dilemma*, p. 48.

46 Ibid., p. 46.

47 Ibid., p. 54.

48 Ibid., p. 23.

49 Ibid., p. 210.

50 Robinson, p. 21.

51 Ibid., p. 41.

52 Pollan, *Omnivore's Dilemma*, p. 84.

53 Shiva, *Stolen Harvest*, p. 27.

54 Manning, *Against the Grain*, p. 124.

55 Ibid., 125.

56 Pyle, p. 17.

57 Resnick.

58 Motavalli.

59 "Agricultural Policy."

60 Ibid.

61 Ibid.

62 Ibid.

63 Murphy et al., p. 8.

64 Ibid., p. 7

65 Weise.

66 Colbert, p. 155.

67 Catton, p. 4.

68 Eades and Eades, *Protein Power LifePlan*, p. 9.

69 Catton, p. xvi.

70 Ibid., p. 27.

71 Ibid., p. 96.

72 Ibid., p. 96.

73 Ibid., p.217.

74 Ibid., p. 28.

75 This phrase is borrowed from the song "The Last Trip Home," by Davy Steele and Alan Reid of Battlefield Band, *Leaving Friday Harbor*, Temple Records, 1999.

76 Catton, *Overshoot*, p. 39.

77 Ibid., p. 39.

78 Ibid., p. 41.

79 Merkel, p. 55.

80 Ibid., p. 58.

81 Ibid., p. 169.

82 Catton, p. 5.

83   McBay.

84   Stoll, p. 17.

85   Merkel, p. 80.

86   Ibid., p. 21.

87   Donahue, p. 218.

88   Donahue, p. 250.

89   Hemenway, p. 6.

90   Allport.

91   Niethammer, p. 208.

92   One example is the New Guinea Baruya, in which young boys were orally raped as part of their initiation away from the world of women and into the world of men. Some young boys resisted until their assailants broke the boys' necks. This resistance was seen as a shameful secret and the victims' bodies were buried without ceremony. Patriarchy would be boring in its sameness if it wasn't so horrible. See Godelier, p. 53. See also Adam, Greenberg, Herdt, Keesing, and W.L. Williams.

93   Altman.

94   See Griffin and Caputi.

95   The wealthier of the Coast Salish, a slave-owning salmon culture of the Pacific Northwest, imprisoned their girl children in so-called "puberty cells," small, dark cages inside the family longhouse, for several years. The girls weren't allowed out during the day, and only occasionally at night. It was essentially footbinding for the whole body. Their bones were so deformed that for the rest of their lives, many of them were unable to walk correctly (Niethammer, p. 41). If women are human, then this is torture (see MacKinnon). Similarly, pubescent girls of the Tlingit, a salmon culture of the Alaskan coast, were isolated in a small room for an entire year, allowed outside only at night and if wearing a broad hat "so as not to taint the stars with her gaze." (Niethammer, p. 39). A woman of the Fox tribe recalls being told, "The state of being a young woman is evil.... Whenever you become a young woman [menstruate] you are to hide yourself." (Ibid., p. 39.) In tribes from the Chickasaw to the Ojibwa, women and girls were expected to isolate themselves away from the tribe during menstruation. In rape cultures, what this meant was that they were exceedingly vulnerable to assault and murder from bands of men, either from their own tribes or from neighboring tribes. (Ibid, pp. 41 and 49.)

96   Ibid., pp. 57-103. Niethammer includes information about the egalitarian cultures of indigenous North America.

97   A Creek man would tie his wife to a tree and shoot her with arrows if he thought she'd been unfaithful. One Gros Ventre man cut off his wife's breasts and arms by way of killing her.(Neithammer, pp. 216-217.) There are accounts of Cherokee men tying their wives to stakes and inviting other men to gang rape her as punishment. The men of the Cheyenne tribe had a similar form of torture called "putting a woman on the prairie," in which a large number of the tribe's men would rape the accused woman. (Ibid., p. 218.) Among the Chipewyan,

"[W]omen were often treated cruelly by their husbands and fathers.... If a woman didn't please her husband in any small way, she could expect a beating, and though it was an odious crime for a Chipewyan male to kill another man, no one thought much about it when a woman died from a beating delivered by her husband. It is no wonder that female infants were often allowed to die of exposure immediately after birth. Chipewyan women considered this practice kind in the long run and were often heard to say that they wished their mothers had done the same for them." (Ibid., p. 131.)

Ojibwa men raped women and girls in their tribe, including in their own households: "It was also common for a man to take his stepdaughter out duck hunting with him and then attempt to rape her while they were away from the village." (Ibid., p. 225.) Among the Yurok of northern California, men considered women "dark, inferior and contaminating." (Ibid., p. 131.) Among the Shoshone, if a woman sat with her legs too far apart it was her male relatives "duty" to shove a burning stick between her thighs. (Ibid., p. 208.) There is no society on earth that has sanctioned women's sadistic control over men's sexuality, let alone with burning sticks on their genitals.

98   Allport, p.197.

99   Ibid., p. 193.

100   Niethammer, p. 131.

101   Ibid., p.194.

102   Mellin et al. See also Maine.

103   "Eating Disorder Statistics."

104   "Statistics," quoting "A report on the behaviour and attitudes of Canadians with respect to weight consciousness and weight control." The Canadian Gallup Poll, Ltd. June 1984.

105   Adolescent Medicine Committee, Canadian Paediatric Society.

106   Cavanaugh.

107 Meanwhile, battering is the most commonly committed violent crime in America: that's a man beating up a woman. And the most likely sexual assailant against a girl is her father or stepfather. From the South American rainforest to the North American suburbs, why is male dominance so endlessly the same?

108 Krech, p. 121.

109 Hemenway, p. 7.

110 Manning, *Against the Grain*, p. 38.

111 Derrick Jensen, p. 17.

112 Manning, p. 33.

113 Manning, p. 71.

114 Manning, p. 72.

115 "100-Watt Virtual People."

116 Manning, p. 45.

117 Manning, p. 48.

Chapter 4

1 Eades and Eades, *Protein Power LifePlan*, p. 7.

2 Ibid., p. 5.

3 Ibid., p. 9.

4 Wolfe, p. 189.

5 Eades and Eades, *Protein Power LifePlan*, p. 3.

6 "Hall of Human Origins."

7 Eades and Eades, *Protein Power LifePlan*, p. 6.

8 Ibid., p. 2.

9 Pitts and Roberts, p. 226.

10 Balzer.

11 Ibid.

12 Cordain, p. 22.

13 Balzer.

14 "Paleo Diet."

15 Eades and Eades, *Protein Power LifePlan*, p. 14.

16 Ibid., p. 14.

17 Ibid., p. 4.

18 Ibid., p. 139.

19 Ibid., p. 141.

20 Ibid., p. 143.

21 Ibid., p. 143.

22 Sullivan.

23 Cordain, p. 46.

24 Daniel, p. 229.

25 Ibid., p. 46.

26 Moral vegetarians take note: this is how similar plants are to us—our own immune systems can't tell us apart.

27 Glucosamine is a dietary supplement taken for arthritis. It works because it inactivates the lectins in wheat, stopping the inflammation they cause in the gut and joints.

28 Eades and Eades, *Protein Power LifePlan*, p 144.

29 Ibid., p. 145.

30 Cordain, p. 57.

31 Ibid., p. 51.

32 Eades and Eades, *Protein Power LifePlan*, p. 145.

33 Eades and Eades, *Protein Power*, p. 8.

34   Eades and Eades, *Protein Power LifePlan*, p .24.

35   Oliver, p. 14.

36   Eades and Eades, *Protein Power*, p. 27.

37   Eades and Eades, *Protein Power LifePlan*, p. 155.

38   Ibid., p. 156.

39   "About Diabetes."

40   Eades and Eades, *Protein Power*, p. 35.

41   Eades and Eades, *Protein Power LifePlan*, p. 160.

42   Ibid., p. 160.

43   Cowan.

44   Colpo, p. 33.

45   Steiner and Kendall, p. 433.

46   Colpo, p. 33.

47   Ibid., p. 34.

48   Jacobs, p. 1046.

49   Colpo, p. 24.

50   Zuriek, p 137-143.

51   Horwich, p. 216.

52   Colpo, p. 54.

53   Yudkin, J., "Diet and coronary thrombosis."

54   Ravnskov, p. 25.

55   Ibid., xxiv.

56   Colpo, p. 38.

57   Kendrick, p.53. For quote, see Colpo, p. 42.

58   Ibid., p. 52.

59   Prentice, p. 6.

60   I realize that using the term "American" to describe people who live in the U.S.A. reflects the entitlement of dominance: Canadians and Mexicans also live in America, as do Nicaraguans and Brazilians. The problem is there's no parallel term—"United Statesian" doesn't exist. In previous chapters, I tried to use constructions like "citizens of the US" and "US American." In this chapter, it's unwieldy to the point of incomprehensibility. I hope someone comes up with a better term soon. Until then, I need the reader to understand me, with apologies.

61   Mann, p. 1.

62   Fallon, *Nourishing Traditions*, p. 246.

63   Schmid, p. 121.

64   Ibid, p. 121.

65   Prior.

66   Kendrick, p. 71.

67   Colpo, p. 50.

68   Ibid., p. 50.

69   Ibid., p. 49.

70   Eades and Eades, *Protein Power LifePlan*, p. xvi.

71   Ibid., p. xvi.

72   Ibid., p. xviii.

73   Ibid., p. xviii.

74   Ibid., p. xx. See for instance the *American Journal of Clinical Nutrition* March 1998 Supplement.

75   Ibid., p. xxi.

76   Colpo, p. 17.

77   Ibid., p. 51.

78   Ibid., p. 60.

79   Ibid., p. 65.

80   See Christakis et al., "Effect of the Anti-Coronary Club Program" and "The Anti-Coronary Club."

81   Fallon, *Nourishing Traditions*, p. 139.

82   Ibid., p. 139.

83   Ibid., p. 9.

84   Enig, p. 71.

85   Ibid., p. 72.

86   Ibid., p. 71.

87   "Rickets." See also Outila and Joiner.

88   Dagnelie et al., "High prevalence of rickets in infants on macrobiotic diets."

89   Enig, p. 50.

90   Ibid., p. 56.

91   Daniel, p. 76.

92   Kendrick, p. 75.

93   Herper.

94   Kendrick, p. 178.

95   Engelberg.

96   Muldoon et al.

97   Golomb.

98   Colpo, p. 26.

99   Ibid., p. 25.

100 Ibid., p. 26.

101 Eades and Eades, *Protein Power LifePlan*, p. 32.

102 Fallon, *Nourishing Traditions*, p. 10.

103 Ibid., p. 10.

104 Fallon, "The Oiling of America."

105 Fallon, *Nourishing Traditions*, p. 11.

106 Ibid., p. 11.

107 "Prostaglandin."

108 Robinson, p. 30.

109 Ibid., p. 31.

110 Fallon, *Nourishing Traditions*, p. 11.

111 Robinson, p. 32.

112 Fallon, *Nourishing Traditions*, p. 5.

113 Ross, *Mood Cure*, p. 129.

114 Price, p. 1. I need to add that as important as his book is, it's also flawed by racism. For instance, his use of the word "primitives" to describe indigenous people is not acceptable to us today. There are other cringe-worthy moments in his book and I don't want to gloss that over. I also believe his project was anti-racist in a larger sense. His underlying thesis, that there is a basic physiological template common to all humans, means that he understood that race is not biologically real, but socially constructed. That idea was and still is progressive. But the book is a product of its time, for better and for worse.

115 Ibid., p. 4.

116 Schmid, *Native Nutrition*, p. 22.

117 Ibid., p. 24.

118 Ibid., p. 25.

119 Ibid., p. 25.

120   Schmid, *Untold Story of Milk*, p. 132.

121   Ibid., p. 136.

122   Sally Fallon, "Ancient Dietary Wisdom."

123   Schmid, *Untold Story of Milk*, p. 108.

124   Ibid., p. 109.

125   Ibid., p. 105.

126   Ibid., p. 106.

127   Ibid., p. 106.

128   Gary Taubes, "What If It's All Been A Big Fat Lie?"

129   Schmid, *Untold Story of Milk*, p. 107.

130   Ibid., p. 136.

131   Price, p. 282.

132   Ross, *Mood Cure*, p. 28.

133   Aric McBay, personal correspondence.

134   Ross, *Mood Cure*, p. 100.

135   Ibid., p. 112.

136   Ibid., p. 27.

137   DeSilver.

138   Apologies to C.S. Lewis.

139   Taubes, *Good Calories, Bad Calories* and Schmid, *Untold Story of Milk*.

140   Schmid, *Untold Story of Milk*, p. 143.

141   Ibid., p. 151.

142   Ibid., p. 152.

143   Taubes, "What If It's All Been A Big Fat Lie?"

144   Schmid, *Untold Story of Milk*, p. 152.

145   Taubes, "What If It's All Been A Big Fat Lie?"

146   Ibid.

147   Ibid.

148   Ibid.

149   Schmid, *Untold Story of Milk*, p. 153.

150   Ibid., p 153.

151   Ibid., p. 149.

152   Ibid., p. 149.

153   Ibid., p. 150.

154   Gary Taubes, *Good Calories, Bad Calories*, p. 5.

155   Ibid., p. 6.

156   Ibid., p. 7. "According to the Bureau of the Census, in 1910, out of every thousand men born in America 250 would die of cardiovascular disease, compared with 110 from degenerative diseases, including diabetes and nephritis; 102 from influenza, pneumonia, and bronchitis; 75 from tuberculosis; and 73 from infections and parasites. Cancer was eighth on the list. By 1950, infectious diseases had been subdued, largely thanks to the discovery of antibiotics: male deaths from pneumonia, influenza, and bronchitis had dropped to 33 per thousand; tuberculosis deaths accounted for only 21; infections and parasites 12. Now cancer was second on the list, accounting for 133 deaths per thousand. Cardiovascular

disease accounted for 560 per thousand."

157 Ibid., p. 8.
158 Ibid., p. 8.
159 Colpo, p. 6.
160 Ibid., p. 7.
161 Sytkowski et al.
162 Colpo, p. 9.
163 Taubes, *Good Calories, Bad Calories*, p. xviii.
164 Ibid., p. xviii.
165 Colpo, p. 7.
166 Taubes, *Good Calories, Bad Calories*, p. xvii.
167 Ibid., p. xviii.
168 Ibid., p. 10.
169 Ibid., p. xix.
170 Ibid., p. xx.
171 Ibid., p. 93.
172 Ibid., p. 94.
173 Ibid., p. 96.
174 Ibid., p. 102.
175 Ibid., p. 103.
176 Ibid., p. 94.
177 Ibid., p. 99.
178 Ibid., p. 98.
179 Ibid., p. 213.
180 Ibid., p. 213.
181 Ibid., p. 190.
182 Ibid., p. 113.
183 Ibid., p. 113.
184 Ibid., p. 159.
185 See for instance, Yudkin.
186 Taubes, *Good Calories, Bad Calories*, p. 45.
187 Ibid., p. 122.
188 Ibid., p. 45.
189 Ibid., p. 47.
190 Ibid., p. 47.
191 Ibid., p. 56.
192 Ibid., p. 27.
193 Ibid., p. 62.
194 Ibid., p. 62.
195 Ibid., p. 72.
196 Ibid., p. 72.
197 Ibid., p. 74.
198 Ibid., p. 74.
199 Ibid., p. 80.
200 Fallon, "Introduction" in Daniel, p. 6.
201 Daniel, p. 9.
202 Ibid., p. 10.
203 Ibid., p. 10.
204 Ibid., p. 13.
205 Manning, *Against the Grain*, p. 71. As discussed in Chapter 3, agriculture produces chronic hunger. Desperate levels of famine in China, for instance, gave rise to the practice of *Yi zi er shi*—"Swop child, make soup." A family would starve one of their daughters and then trade her body for a neighbor's dead girl to use for food. And it was, of course, always girls. See Dworkin, *Scapegoat*, p. 12, for more on transcultural female starvation. See also my discussion in Chapter 3.
206 Ibid., p. 314.
207 Ibid., p. 314.

208 Ibid., p. 318.

209 Ibid., p. 320.

210 Ibid., p. 321.

211 Ibid., p. 321.

212 Ibid., p. 357.

213 Ibid., p. 357.

214 Ibid., p. 359.

215 Ibid., p. 298.

216 Ibid., p. 359.

217 Ibid., p. 361.

218 Ibid., p. 364.

219 She has since had to have a hysterectomy. You're allowed to learn from her mistake.

220 Ibid., p. 361.

221 Ibid., p. 386.

222 Ibid., p. 368.

223 Ibid., p. 364.

224 Ibid., p. 307.

225 Ibid., p. 308.

226 Ibid., p. 308.

227 Ibid., p. 308.

228 Ibid., p. 350.

229 Ibid., p. 350.

230 Ibid., p. 353.

231 Ibid., p. 353.

232 Ibid., p. 334.

233 Ibid., p. 331.

234 Ibid., p. 332.

235 Ibid., p. 372.

236 Ibid., p. 373.

237 Fallon and Enig, "Caustic Commentary Spring 2000."

238 "Frequently Asked Questions about WIC."

239 "Breastfeeding."

240 "Nestlé Boycott."

241 See Baby Milk Action to get involved. http://www.babymilkaction.org/

242 The exception being Sally Fallon, president of the Weston A. Price Foundation (see especially Fallon, "Foundation Testimony"), and Kaayla Daniel, author of *The Whole Soy Story*.

243 Fallon and Enig, "Tragedy & Hype."

244 Fallon, "Introduction," p. 2.

245 Daniel, p. 63. See also "Sales and Trends."

246 Daniel, p. 66.

247 Ibid., p. 67.

248 Ibid., p. 69.

249 Ibid., p. 69.

250 Ibid., p. 90.

251 Ibid., p. 92.

252 Ibid., p. 93.

253 Ibid., p. 93

254 Ibid., p. 95.

255 Ibid., p. 124.

256 Ibid., p. 125.

257 Ibid., p. 127.

258 Ibid., p. 128.

259 Ibid., p. 28.

260 Ibid., p. 28.

261 Fallon and Enig, "Soy: The Dark Side."

262 Ibid., p. 15.

263 Ibid., p. 369.

264 Ibid., p. 148.

265 Quoted in Daniel, p. 343.

266 "Late Breaking News."

267 Barclay and Vega.

268 Daniel, p. 31.

269 Quoted in Daniel, p. 365.

270 Krizmanic.

271 Ross, *Mood Cure,* p. 45.

272 Wolf, p. 187.

273 Hornbacher, p. 217.

274 Ross, *Diet Cure,* p. 23.

275 Ibid., p. 33.

276 Ibid., p. 24.

277 Ibid., p. 25.

278 Ibid., p. 33.

279 Ibid., p. 23.

280 Ross, *Mood Cure*, p. 28.

281 Hornbacher, p. 245.

282 Bratman.

283 Nicholson.

284 Hawkes.

285 Puotinen, p. 50, quoting a study in the medical journal *Human Reproduction* of 8,000 infants.

286 See for instance the case of a thirty-three-year-old vegan who permanently damaged his eye sight. Mercola, "Strict Vegetarians Can Develop Blindness and Brain Damage."

287 Mercola, "Vegetarian Diet Increases Alzheimer's Risk" and "Vegetarian Diet Can Cause Repeat Miscarriages."

288 "Neurologic Impairment in Children Associated with Maternal Dietary Deficiency of Cobalamin."

289 Fallon and Enig, "Caustic Commentary," quoting from Science News Online, 12/23-30/2000, Vol. 158, No 26-27.

290 Dagnelie et al., "Effects of macrobiotic diets on linear growth."

291 Roberts.

292 Brody.

293 Keddy.

294 Mercoal, "Dangers of a Vegetarian Diet in Teens."

295 Colpo, p. 299.

296 According to Steven Aldana, "Longitudinal studies of these vegetarians [SDAs] revealed that men in this group lived 7.3 years longer than the national average and the women lived 4.4 years longer. Those who also exercised, avoided tobacco use, and maintained a healthy body weight lived 10 years longer than average. Mormons in the state of California who exercised regularly, did not smoke, and got adequate sleep had death rates due to cancer and cardiovascular disease that were 70–80% lower than the rest of the nation. Males in this population lived an average of 11 years longer than comparable US males, and females lived 7 years longer. By avoiding tobacco use, exercising regularly, and getting enough sleep, these Mormons demonstrated some of the lowest

death rates ever published." See Aldana, p. 4. The references he sites are: Fraser and Shavlik, Fontaine, and Enstrom.

297 Fallon and Enig, *Nourishing Traditions*, p. 253.

298 Byrnes.

299 Key.

Chapter 5

1 Stoll, p. 15.

2 Stamets.

3 Stoll, p. 31.

4 Leu.

5 Bane, p. 57.

6 Ibid.

7 Ruddiman.

8 Donahue.

9 Barlow.

10 Ted Williams, "Horse Sense," p. 36.

11 Ibid., p. 40.

12 See Caufield, especially Chapter 7.

13 Catton, p. 31

14 Kunstler, "Speech to Second Vermont Republic." See also Kunstler, *The Long Emergency*.

15 Heinberg, p. 121.

16 Cordain, p. 24.

17 Catton, p. 186.

18 Heinberg, p. 175.

19 Ibid., p. 121-123.

20 Eisler.

21 Griffin.

22 Grossman.

23 Encyclopedia.com.

24 Gilligan and Spender.

25 Robert Jensen, p. 5.

26 Lenskyj.

27 Langford and Thompson, p. 7.

28 DeKeseredy and Kelly.

29 "UN calls for strong action to eliminate violence against women."

30 Jeffreys, *Industrial*.

31 Dines and Jensen.

32 Jeffreys, "Sado-Masochism," p. 65.

33 Derrick Jensen, p. 342.

34 Vidal, "At Home, 1988," p. 334.

35 Buhner, p. 281.

36 Dworkin, "Woman-Hating Right and Left," p. 30.

37 Brody, p. 85.

38 Derrick Jensen.

Bibliography

"100-Watt Virtual People." *Virtual People.* http://www.esva.net/~flash/vp.htm (accessed on November 22, 2007).

"2002 Fish Die-Off Facts & Articles." *Our Klamath Basin Water Crisis.* http://www. klamathforestalliance.org (accessed on July 3, 2007).

"About Diabetes." *Defeat Diabetes Foundation.* http://www.defeatdiabetes.org/ aboutdiabetes.htm (accessed on July 15, 2007).

Adam, B.D. "Age, Structure, and Sexuality: Reflections on the Anthropological Evidence on Homosexual Relations." *Journal of Homosexuality* 11, 1985: pp. 19-33.

Adolescent Medicine Committee, Canadian Paediatric Society, "Eating Disorders in Adolescents: Principles of Diagnosis and Treatment." *Paediatrics and Child Health* 3, no. 3, 1998: pp. 189-92.

"Agricultural Policy." *Wikipedia.* http://en.wikipedia.org/wiki/Agricultural_policy# Dumping_is_harmful_to_developing_world_farmers (accessed on April 3, 2007).

Aldana, Steven G. *The Culprit and the Cure: Why Lifestyle Is the Culprit Behind America's Poor Health and How Transforming That Lifestyle Can Be the Cure.* North Mapleton, UT: Maple Mountain Press, 2005.

Allport, Susan. *The Primal Feast: Food, Sex, Foraging and Love.* New York: Harmony Books, 2000.

Altman, Lawrence K. "Women Worldwide Nearing Higher Rate for AIDS Than Men." The New York Times, July 21, 1992, p. C3.

Åredale, Tord. "Why Become a Fruitarian?" *Fruitarian Universal Network*. http://hem.fyristorg.com/fruitarian/why.html (accessed March 27, 2007).

"Bacteria and Human Body Weight." *Google Answers*. http://answers.google.com/answers/threadview?id=208733 (accessed on December 17, 2007).

Balzer, Dr. Ben. "Introduction to the Paleolithic Diet." www.earth360.com/diet_paleodiet_balzer.html (accessed on April 14, 2007).

Bane, Peter. "Storing Carbon in Soil: The Possibilities of a New American Agriculture." *Permaculture Activist*, no. 65, Autumn 2007.

Barclay, Laurie and Charles Vega. "American Heart Association Does Not Recommend Isoflavone Supplements." *Medscape Medical News*. http://www.medscape.com/viewarticle/522256 (accessed on August 23, 2007).

Barlow, Connie. *The Ghosts of Evolution: Nonsensical Fruit, Missing Partners, and Other Ecological Anachronisms*. New York: Basic Books, 2002.

Berry, Thomas. "Forward," in Joanne Elizabeth Lauck, *The Voice of the Infinite in the Small: Re-Visioning the Insect-Human Connection*. Boston: Shambhala, 2002.

"Breastfeeding: Some Strategies Used to Market Infant Formula May Discourage Breastfeeding; State Contracts Should Better Protect against Misuse of WIC Name." *United States Government Accountability Office*. http://www.gao.gov/new.items/d06282.pdf (accessed on October 17, 2007).

Bratman, Steven. "Health Food Junkie." *Yoga Journal*. October 1997. http://www.beyondveg.com/bratman-s/hfj/hf-junkie-1a.shtml (accessed on December 11, 2007).

Brody, Hugh. *The Other Side of Eden*. New York: North Point Press, 2000.

Brody, Jane. "Personal Health." *The New York Times*. March 15, 1987. http://query.nytimes.com/gst/fullpage.html?res=9B0DE4D91F3EF936A15750C0A9619 48260&sec=health&spon=&pagewanted=1 (accessed December 3, 2009).

Brumberg, Joan Jackson. *Fasting Girls: The History of Anorexia Nervosa*. New York: Penguin Books, 1988.

Bruhner, Stephen Harrod. *The Lost Language of Plants: The Ecological Importance of Plant Medicines to Life on Earth*. White River Junction, VT: Chelsea Green, 2002.

Byrnes, Stephen. "Are Saturated Fats Really Dangerous For You?" http://www.mercola.com/2002/feb/23/vegetarianism_myths_06.htm

Caputi, Jane. *Gossips, Gorgons & Crones: The Fates of the Earth*. Santa Fe, NM: Bear & Company Publishing, 1993.

Catton, William R. *Overshoot: The Ecological Basis of Revolutionary Change*. Urbana: University of Illinois Press, 1980.

Caufield, Catherine. *In the Rainforest: Report from a Strange, Beautiful, Imperiled World*. Chicago: University of Chicago Press, 1991.

Cavanaugh, Carolyn, "What We Know About Eating Aisorders: Facts and Statistics." In Lemberg, Raymond and Cohn, Leigh, eds., *Eating Disorders: A Reference Sourcebook*. Phoenix, AZ: Oryx Press, 1999.

G. Christakis, S. H. Rinzler, M. Archer, and A. Kraus. "Effect of the Anti-Coronary Club Program on Coronary Heart Disease. Risk Factor Status." *JAMA* 198, no. 6, Nov. 7, 1966: pp. 597-604.

-----"The Anti-Coronary Club: A Dietary Approach to the Prevention of Coronary Heart Disease—a Seven-Year Report." *American Journal of Public Health and the Nation's Health* 56, no. 2, Feb. 1966: pp. 299-314.

Colbert, Elizabeth. *Field Notes from a Catastrophe: Man, Nature and Climate Change*. New York: Bloomsbury Publishing, 2006.

Colpo, Anothony. *The Great Cholesterol Con: Why Everything You've Been Told About Cholesterol, Diet and Heart Disease Is Wrong!* Lulu, 2006.

Cordain, Loren. "Cereal Grains: Humanity's Double-Edged Sword." In Artemis P. Simopoulos, ed., *Evolutionary Aspects of Nutrition and Health: Diet, Exercise, Genetics and Chronic Disease (World Review of Nutrition and Dietetics) (v. 84)*. Basel, Switzerland: S. Karger Publishers, 1999.

Cowan, Tom. "Ask the Doctor About Gastroparesis." http://www.westonaprice. org/askdoctor/gastroparesis.html (accessed on September 25, 2007).

Dagnelie, P.C., M. van Dusseldorp, W.A. van Staveren and J.G.A.J. Hautvast. "Effects of macrobiotic diets on linear growth in infants and children until 10 years of age." Department of Human Nutrition, Agricultural University Wageningen, Wageningen, The Netherlands. http://www.unu.edu/unupress/ food2/UID06E/uid06e0p.htm (acccessed on April 7, 2007).

Dagnelie P.C., J.V.R.A. Vergote, W.A. van Staveren WA. "High Prevalence of Rickets in Infants on Macrobiotic Diets." *American Journal of Clinical Nutrition* 51, 1990: pp. 201-208.

Daniel, Kaayla T. *The Whole Soy Story: The Dark Side of America's Favorite Health Food*. Washington, D.C.: New Trends Publishing, Inc., 2005.

DeKeseredy, W. and K. Kelly. "The Incidence and Prevalence of Woman Abuse in Canadian University and College Dating Relationships: Results From a National Survey." Ottawa: Health Canada, 1993.

DeSilver, Drew. "Putting Meat Back on Their Menu." *Vegetarian Times*, January 1995. http://findarticles.com/p/articles/mi_m0820/is_n209/ai_15982870/ pg_1 (accessed June 113, 2007).

Dines, Gail and Robert Jensen. "Pornography Is A Left Issue." *ZNet*. http://www.zmag.org/content/showarticle.cfm?ItemID=9272 (accessed on December 13, 2007).

Donahue, Brian. *Reclaiming the Commons: Community Farms and Forests in a New England Town.* New Haven: Yale University Press, 2001.

Dworkin, Andrea. *Scapegoat: The Jews, Israel, and Women's Liberation.* New York: The Free Press, 2000.

----"Woman-Hating Right and Left." In *The Sexual Liberals and the Attack on Feminism,* Dorchen Leidholdt and Janice G. Raymond, eds. New York: Teachers College Press, 1990.

Eades, Michael R., M.D., and Mary Dan Eades, M.D. *Protein Power.* New York: Bantam Books, 1999.

----*The Protein Power LifePlan.* New York: Warner Books, 2000.

"Eating Disorder Statistics." *Eating Disorders Coalition.* http://www. eatingdisorderscoalition.org/documents/Statistics_000.pdf (accessed on May 7, 2007).

Eisler, Riane. *The Chalice and the Blade: Our History, Our Future.* New York: HarperCollins, 1987.

Ekarius, Carol. *Small Scale Livestock Farming: A Grass-Based Approach for Health, Sustainability, and Profit.* North Adams, Massachusetts: Storey Books, 1999.

Enig, Mary. *Know Your Fats: The Complete Primer for Understanding the Nutrition of Fats, Oils and Cholesterol.* Bethesda: Bethesda Press, 2000.

Engelberg, H. "Low Serum Cholesterol and Suicide." *Lancet,* no. 339, March 21, 1992: pp. 727-728.

Enstrom, J.E. "Health Practices and Cancer Mortality Among Active California Mormons." *Journal of the National Cancer Institute* 81, no. 23, Dec 6, 1989: pp. 1807–14.

Fallon, Sally. "Ancient Dietary Wisdom for Tomorrow's Children." *Weston A. Price Foundation.* http://www.westonaprice.org/traditional_diets/ancient_dietary_ wisdom.html (accessed on October 14, 2007).

----"Foundation Testimony on Federal Policies." *Weston A. Price Foundation.* http:// www.westonaprice.org/federalupdate/testimony/testimony.html (accessed on July 16, 2007).

----"Introduction." In Kaayla T. Daniel, *The Whole Soy Story: The Dark Side of America's Favorite Health Food* (Washington, D.C.: New Trends Publishing, Inc., 2005.

Fallon, Sally and Mary Enig. "Caustic Commentary Spring 2000." *Weston A. Price Foundation* http://www.westonaprice.org/causticcommentary/cc2000sp.html (accessed on September 4, 2007).

----"Caustic Commentary Summer 2003." *Weston A. Price Foundation.* http://www. westonaprice.org/causticcommentary/cc2003su.html.

----*Nourishing Traditions.* Washington, D.C.: New Trends Publishing, 2001.

----"The Oiling of America." http://www.westonaprice.org/knowyourfats/oiling. html#40 (accessed on June 3, 2007).

----"Soy: The Dark Side of America's Favorite 'Health' Food." http://www. westonaprice.org/soy/darkside.html (accessed on August 23, 2007).

----"Tragedy & Hype: The Third International Soy Symposium." http://www. westonaprice.org/soy/tragedy.html (accessed on August 23, 2007).

Ferber, Dan. "Duck Soup," *Audubon* 108, no.3, May-June 2006.

Fontaine, K.R., D.T. Redden, C. Wang, A.O. Westfall, and D.B. Allison. "Years of Life Lost Due to Obesity." *Journal of the American Medical Association* 289, no. 2, January 8, 2003: pp. 187–93.

Fraser, G.E. and D.J. Shavlik. "Ten Years of Life: Is It a Matter of Choice?" *Archives of Internal Medicine* 161, no. 13, July 9, 2001: pp. 1645–52.

"Frequently Asked Questions about WIC." *USDA Food and Nutrition Service.* http://www.fns.usda.gov/wic/FAQs/faq.htm#8 (accessed on August 11, 2007).

Gilligan, Carol. *In a Different Voice.* Cambridge: Harvard University Press, 1982.

----*Making Connections: The Relational Worlds of Adolescent Girls at Emma Willard School.* Cambridge: Harvard University Press, 1990.

Godelier, Maurice. *The Making of Great Men: Male Domination and Power among the New Guinea Baruya.* Cambridge, England: Cambridge University Press, 1986.

Golomb, B.A. "Cholesterol and Violence: Is There a Connection?" *Annals of Internal Medicine* 128, 1998: pp. 478-487.

Greenberg, D. *The Construction of Homosexuality.* Chicago: University of Chicago Press, 1988.

Griffin, Susan. *Pornography and Silence: Culture's Revenge Against Nature.* New York: Harper & Row, Publishers, 1981.

----*Woman and Nature: The Roaring Inside Her.* New York: HarperCollins, 1979.

Grossman, Lt. Col. Dave. *On Killing: The Psychological Cost of Learning to Kill in War and Society.* New York: Little, Brown and Company, 1995.

"Hall of Human Origins." *American Museum of Natural History.* http://www.amnh. org/exhibitions/permanent/humanorigins/human/art.php (accessed on April 12, 2007).

Hawkes, Nigel. "Low-fat food is 'bad for you.'" *The Times,* February 28, 2007.

Heinberg, Richard. *Peak Everything: Waking Up To the Century of Declines.* Gabriola Island, BC: New Society, 2007.

Heitschmidt, Rodney K. and Jerry W. Stuth, eds. *Grazing Management: An Ecological Perspective.* Portland, OR: Timber Press, 1991.

Hemenway, Toby. "Is Sustainable Agriculture an Oxymoron?" *Permaculture Activist* 60, May 2006.

Herdt, G. "Representations of Homosexuality: An Essay on Cultural Ontology and Historical Comparison (Part I)." *Journal of the History of Sexuality* 1, 1991.

----"Representations of Homosexuality: An Essay on Cultural Ontology and Historical Comparison (Part II)." *Journal of the History of Sexuality* 1, 1991.

---- *The Sambia: Ritual and gender in New Guinea.* New York: Harcourt Brace Jovanovich, 1987.

Herper, Matthew and Peter Kang. "The World's Ten Best-Selling Drugs." *Forbes*, March 22, 2006. http://www.forbes.com/2006/03/21/pfizer-merck-amgen-cx_mh_pk_0321topdrugs.html (accessed on November 4, 2007).

Hillel, Daniel. *Out of the Earth: Civilization and the Life of the Soil.* New York: The Free Press, 1991.

Hochschild, Adam. *Bury the Chains: Prophets and Rebels in the Fight to Free an Empire's Slaves.* New York: Houghton Mifflin, 2005.

Hornbacher, Marya. *Wasted: A Memoir of Anorexia and Bulimia.* New York: Harper Perennial, 1999.

Horwich, T.B., M.A. Hamilton, and G.C. Fonarow . "Low Serum Cholesterol Is Associated with Marked Increase in Mortality in Advanced Heart Failure." *Journal of Cardiac Failure* 8, no. 4, 2002: pp. 216-224.

"Inedia." *Wikipedia.* http://en.wikipedia.org/wiki/Inedia (accessed on July 16, 2007).

Jackson, Wes. *New Roots for Agriculture.* Lincoln, NE: University of Nebraska Press, 1981.

Jacobs D., et al. "Report of the Conference on Low Blood Cholesterol: Mortality Associations." *Circulation* 86, no. 3, September 1992: pp. 1046-60.

Jeffreys, Sheila. *The Industrial Vagina: The Political Economy of the Global Sex Trade.* London: Routledge, 2008.

----"Sado-Masochism: The Erotic Cult of Fascism." *Lesbian Ethics* 2, No. 1, Spring 1986.

Jensen, Derrick. *Endgame.* New York: Seven Stories Press, 2006.

Jensen, Robert. *Getting Off: Pornography and the End of Masculinity.* Boston: South End Press, 2007.

Joiner, Terence A., Carol Foster, and Thomas Shope. "The Many Faces of Vitamin D Deficiency Rickets." *Pediatrics in Review* 21, no. 9, 2000: pp. 296-302.

Keddy, Diane. "Nutrition Hotline." *Eating Disorders Today* 1, no. 2, Spring 2002. http://www.gurze.com/client/client_pages/newsletteredt5.cfm (accessed on November 25, 2007).

Keesing, R.M. "Prologue: Toward a Multidimensional Understanding of Male Initiation." In G. Herdt, ed., *Rituals of Manhood: Male initiation in Papua New Guinea*. Berkeley, CA: University of California Press, 1982.

Kemmerer, Lisa. "Hunting Tradition: Treaties, Law, and Subsistence Killing," http://www.animalliberationfront.com/Practical/Fishing--Hunting/Hunting/ Hunting%20Tradition.htm (accessed on August 14, 2007).

Kendrick, Dr. Malcolm. *The Great Cholesterol Con: The Truth About What Really Causes Heart Disease and How To Avoid It*. London: John Blake Publishing Ltd., 2007.

Key, T.J., M. Thorogood, P.N. Appleby, and M.L. Burr. "Dietary Habits and Mortality in 11,000 Vegetarians and Non-vegetarians: Detailed Findings from a Collaborative Analysis of 5 Prospective Studies." *British Medical Journal*, no. 313, 1996: pp. 775-9.

"Keystone Species." *Wikipedia*. en.wikipedia.org/wiki/Keystone_species (accessed on November 12, 2008).

Krech, Shepard. *The Ecological Indian: Myth and History*. New York: W.W. Norton & Co., Inc., 1999.

Kunstler, James Howard. *The Long Emergency: Surviving the End of Oil, Climate Change, and Other Converging Catastrophes of the Twenty-First Century*. New York: Grove Press, 2006.

----"Speech to Second Vermont Republic." http://www.kunstler.com/spch_ Vermont%20Oct%2005.htm (accessed December 14, 2007).

Krizmanic, Judy. "Prisoners of the Plate: Can a Meatless Diet Mask an Eating Disorder?" *Vegetarian Times*, April 1995. http://findarticles.com/p/articles/ mi_m0820/is_n212/ai_16845854 (accessed on November 8, 2007).

Langford, Rae and June D. Thompson. *Mosby's Handbook of Diseases, 3rd Edition*. St. Louis, MO: Elsevier Health Sciences, 2005.

"Late Breaking News: Soy Warning from German Consumer Watchdog Organization." *Wise Traditions* 8, no. 4, Winter 2007: p. 64.

Lappé, Frances Moore. *Diet for a Small Planet, 10th Anniversary Edition*. New York: Ballantine Books, 1982.

Lauck, Joanne Elizabeth. *The Voice of the Infinite in the Small: Re-Visioning the Insect-Human Connection*. Boston: Shambhala, 2002.

Lenskyj, Helen. "An Analysis of Violence Against Women: A Manual for Educators and Administrators." Toronto: Ontario Institute for Studies in Education, 1992.

Leu, Andre. "Organic Agriculture Can Feed the World." *Acres USA* 34, no. 1, January 2004.

"Loblolly Marsh Wetland Preserve." *Limberlost Swamp Dedication Celebration.* http://www.tentativetimes.net/porter/dedicate.html (accessed on July 23, 2007).

Lozier, John, Edward Rayburn, and Jane Shaw. "Growing and Selling Pasture-Finished Beef: Results of a Nationwide Survey." *Journal of Sustainable Agriculture.* http://www.wvu.edu/~agexten/forglvst/PFBSurvey.pdf (accessed on June 8, 2007).

Mackie, Roderick I. "Mutualistic Fermentative Digestion in the Gastrointestinal Tract: Diversity and Evolution." *Integrative and Comparative Biology* 42, no. 2, 2002: pp. 319-326. http://icb.oxfordjournals.org/cgi/content/full/42/2/319 (accessed April 23, 2007).

MacKinnon, Catharine. *Are Women Human? And Other International Dialogues.* Cambridge, MA: The Belknap Press of Harvard University Press, 2006.

Maine, Margo. *Body Wars: Making Peace with Women's Bodies.* Carlsbad, CA: Gürze Books, 2000.

"Malaria Facts/CDC Malaria." *Centers for Disease Control and Prevention.* http://www.cdc.gov/malaria/facts.htm (accessed on June 14, 2007).

Malmstrom, Frederick V. "Close Encounters of the Facial Kind." *Skeptic.* http://www.skeptic.com/the_magazine/featured_articles/v11n4_alien_faces.html (accessed on April 8, 2007).

Mann, George V., ed. *Coronary Heart Disease: The Dietary Sense and Nonsense.* London: Veritas Society, 1993.

Manning, Richard. *Against the Grain: How Agriculture Has Hijacked Civilization.* New York: North Point Press, 2004.

----"The Oil We Eat: Following the Food Chain Back to Iraq," *Harper's,* February 2004.

Margulis, Lynn and Dorion Sagan. *What Is Life?* New York: Simon and Schuster, 1995.

McBay, Aric. "An Interview with George Draffan." *In the Wake.* http://www.inthewake.org/draffan1.html (accessed on December 11, 2007).

Mellin, L.M, S. Scully and C.E. Irwin. Paper presented at American Dietetic Assoc. Annual Meeting, October 1986. *National Eating Disorder Information Center.* http://www.nedic.ca/knowthefacts/statistics.shtml (accessed June 15, 2007).

Merchant, Carolyn. *The Death of Nature: Women, Ecology, and the Scientific Revolution.* New York: HarperOne, 1990.

Mercola, Joseph. "Dangers of a Vegetarian Diet in Teens." *Mercola.com.* http://articles.mercola.com/sites/articles/archive/2001/12/29/vegetarian-part-two.aspx (accessed on December 17, 2007).

----"Strict Vegetarians Can Develop Blindness and Brain Damage." *Mercola.com.* http://www.mercola.com/2000/mar/26/vegetarians_blindness.htm (accessed on December 29, 2006).

----Vegetarian Diet Can Cause Repeat Miscarriages." *Mercola.com.* http://www.mercola.com/2001/may/12/vitamin_b12.htm (accessed on September 29, 2007).

----"Vegetarian Diet Increases Alzheimer's Risk." *Mercola.com.* http://articles.mercola.com/sites/articles/archive/2001/05/19/alzheimers-part-three.aspx (accessed on September 29, 2007).

Merkel, Jim. *Radical Simplicity: Small Footprints on a Finite Earth.* Gabriola Island, B.C.: New Society Publishers, 2003.

Mollison, Bill. *Permaculture: A Designer's Manual.* Tyalgum, NSW: Tagari Publications, 1988.

Motavalli, Jim. "So You're an Environmentalist; Why Are You Still Eating Meat?" *E Magazine.* http://www.alternet.org/story/121162/ (accessed on October 28, 2006).

Muldoon, M.F., S.M. Manuck, and K.M. Matthews. "Lowering cholesterol concentrations and mortality: a quantitative review of primary prevention trials." *British Medical Journal,* no. 301., 1990: pp. 309-314.

Murphy, Sophia, Ben Lilliston, and Mary Beth Lake. *WTO Agreement on Agriculture: A Decade of Dumping.* Minneapolis, MN: The Institute for Agriculture and Trade Policy, 2005.

"Nestlé Boycott." *Wikipedia.* http://en.wikipedia.org/wiki/Nestl%C3%A9_boycott (accessed on July 11, 2007).

"Neurologic Impairment in Children Associated with Maternal Dietary Deficiency of Cobalamin." *Morbidity and Mortality Weekly Report* 52, 2003: pp. 61-64. http://www.cdc.gov/mmwr/preview/mmwrhtml/mm5204a1.htm (accessed on April 12, 2007).

Nicholson, Ward. "Paleolithic Diet vs. Vegetarianism: What Was Humanity's Original, Natural Diet?" *Beyond Vegetarianism.* http://www.beyondveg.com/nicholson-w/hb/hb-interview1a.shtml (accessed on November 12, 2007).

Niethammer, Carolyn. *Daughters of the Earth.* New York: Collier Books, 1977.

Oliver, Mary. "Wild Geese." *Dream Work.* New York: Atlantic Monthly Press, 199

Outila, T.A., M.U. Kärkkäinen, R.H. Seppänen, and C.J. Lamberg-Allardt. "Dietary Intake of Vitamin D in Premenopausal, Healthy Vegans Was Insufficient to Maintain Concentrations of Serum 25-Hydroxyvitamin D and Intact Parathyroid Hormone within Normal Ranges During the Winter in Finland." *Journal of American Dietetic Association* 100, no. 4, April 2000: pp. 434-41.

"The Paleo Diet." *The Paleo Diet.* http://www.thepaleodiet.com (accessed on June 12, 2007).

Patzin, Patrisia Gonzales. "Corn Is Our Parent and Elder." http://hometown.aol. com/xcolumn/myhomepage/ (accessed on October 23, 2007).

Paulson, Tom. "The Lowdown on Topsoil: It's Disappearing."*Seattle Post Intelligencer*, Tuesday, January 22, 2008. http://seattlepi.nwsource.com/ local/348200_dirt22.html (accessed February 2, 2008).

Pearce, Fred. *When the Rivers Run Dry: Water—The Defining Crisis of the Twenty-first Century.* Boston: Beacon Press, 2006.

Phillips, Michael. *The Apple Grower: A Guide for the Organic Orchardist.* White River Junction, VT: Chelsea Green Publishing Company, 1998.

Pitts, Michael and Mark Roberts, *Fairweather Eden.* New York: Fromm International, 1997.

Pollan, Michael. *The Botany of Desire.* New York: Random House, 2001.

-----*The Omnivore's Dilemma: A Natural History of Four Meals.* New York: Penguin Press, 2006.

"Prairies of Illinois." *Illinois Department of Natural Resources.* http://dnr.state.il.us/ conservation/naturalheritage/florafauna/document.htm (accessed on June 14, 2007).

Prechtel, Martin. *Long Life, Honey in the Heart.* New York: Thorsons, 2002.

Prentice, Jessica. *Full Moon Feast: Food and the Hunger for Connection.* White River Junction, VT: Chelsea Green Publishing Company, 2006.

Price, Douglas T., and Anne Birgitte Gebauer. *Last Hunters, First Farmers.* Santa Fe: School of American Research Press, 1995.

Price, Weston A. *Nutrition and Physical Degeneration.* La Mesa, CA: The Price-Pottenger Nutritional Foundation, 2000.

Prior, I.A., F. Davidson F, C.E. Salmond, and Z. Czochanska. "Cholesterol, Coconuts, and Diet on Polynesian Atolls: A Natural Experiment: the Pukapuka and Tokelau Island Studies." *American Journal of Clinical Nutrition* 34, no. 8, August 1981: pp. 1552-1561.

"Prostaglandin." *Wikipedia.* http://en.wikipedia.org/wiki/Prostaglandin#Function (accessed on November 13, 2007).

Puotinen, C.J. "Food and Fertility: What You Need To Know Before You Conceive." *Taste For Life*, October 2002.

Purdy, Mark. "The Vegan Ecological Wasteland." http://www.westonaprice.org/ farming/wasteland.html (accessed July 29, 2007).

Pyle, George. *Raising Less Corn, More Hell: The Case for the Independent Farm and Against Industrial Food.* New York: Public Affairs, 2005.

Resnick, Carole. "What We Need to Know about the Corporate Takeover of the 'Organic' Food Market." http://www.peacecouncil.net/pnl/03/718/718CorporateTakeover.htm (accessed on August 3, 2007).

"Rickets." *Nutrition and Well-Being A to Z.* http://www.faqs.org/nutrition/Pre-Sma/Rickets.html (accessed on November 17, 2007).

Rindos, David. *Origins of Agriculture: An Evolutionary Perspective.* New York: Academic Press, 1984.

Ravnskov, Uffe. *The Cholesterol Myths.* Washington, DC: New Trends Publishing, 2000.

"A Report on the Behaviour and Attitudes of Canadians with Respect to Weight Consciousness and Weight Control." The Canadian Gallup Poll, Ltd. June 1984. *www.nedic.ca/knowthefacts/statistics.shtml (accessed on July 23, 2007).*

Roberts, Michelle. "Children 'Harmed' by Vegan Diets." *BBC News*, February 21, 2005, http://news.bbc.co.uk/2/hi/health/4282257.stm (accessed on December 3, 2007).

Robinson, Jo. *Pasture Perfect: The Far-Reaching Benefits of Choosing Meat, Eggs, and Dairy Products from Grass-Fed Animals.* Vashon, WA: Vashon Island Press, 2004.

Roosevelt, Theodore. *African Game Trails: An Account of the African Wanderings of an American Hunter-Naturalist.* New York: St. Martin's Press, 1988.

Ross, Julia. *The Diet Cure,* New York: Viking, 1999.

---- *The Mood Cure.* New York: Viking, 2002.

Ruddiman, William F. *Plows, Plagues, and Petroleum: How Humans Took Control of Climate.* Princeton: Princeton University Press, 2005.

Sahlins, Marshall. *Stone Age Economics.* Piscataway, NJ: Aldine Transactions, 1972.

Salatin, Joel. "Balance: Stability for Your Life and Farm." *Acres USA* 34, no. 1, January 2004.

Schmid, Ron. *Native Nutrition: Eating According to Ancestral Wisdom.* Rochester, VT: Healing Arts Press, 1994.

---- *The Untold Story of Milk: Green Pastures, Contented Cows and Raw Dairy Foods.* Washington, DC: New Trends Publishing, 2003.

Scrunton, Roger. *Animal Rights and Wrongs.* London: Claridge Press Ltd, 1996.

Shenk, Joshua Wolf. *Lincoln's Melancholy: How Depression Challenged a President and Fueled His Greatness. New York:* Houghton Mifflin, 2005.

Shiva, Vandana. *Stolen Harvest: The Hijacking of the Global Food Supply.* London: Zed Books, 2000.

Siegel, Robert. "Exploring Lincoln's Melancholy." *NPR.* www.npr.org/templates/story/story.php?storyId=4976127 (accessed on October 13, 2007).

"Sales and Trends." *Soyfoods Association of North America*. http://www.soyfoods.org/ products/sales-and-trends/ (accessed on September 18, 2007).

Spender, Dale. *Invisible Women: The Schooling Scandal*. London: Readers and Writers Publishing Cooperative, 1982.

Stamets, Paul. *Mycelium Running: How Mushrooms Can Help Save the World*. Berkeley, CA: Ten Speed Press, 2005.

"Statistics." *National Eating Disorder Information Center*. http://www.nedic.ca/ knowthefacts/statistics.shtml (accessed June 15, 2007).

Steckel, Richard H., and Jerome C. Rose. "Introduction." *The Backbone of History*. New York: Cambridge University Press, 2002.

Steiner, A., and F.E. Kendall F.E. "Atherosclerosis and Arteriosclerosis in Dogs Following Ingestion of Cholesterol and Thiouracil." *Archives of Pathology* 42, 1946.

Stoll, Steven. *Larding the Lean Earth: Soil and Society in Nineteenth-Century America*. New York: Hill and Wang, 2002.

Stout, Ruth. *The Ruth Stout No-Work Garden Book*. Emmaeus, PA: Rodale Press, 1971.

"The Struggle to Save Salmon in the Klamath Basin." *The Pacific Coast Federtion of Fishermen's Association*. http://www.pcffa.org/klamath.htm (accessed on June 27, 2007).

Sullivan, Krispin. "The Lectin Report." *The Lectin Story*. www.krispin.com/lectin. html (accessed on June 23, 2007).

"Swainson's Warbler." *Cornell Lab of Ornithology All About Birds*. http://www.birds. cornell.edu/ (accessed on July 16, 2007).

Sytkowski, P.A., W.B. Kannel, and R.B. D'Agostino. "Changes in Risk Factors and the Decline in Mortality from Cardiovascular Disease. The Framingham Study." *New England Journal of Medicine* 332, no.23, June 7, 1990: pp. 1635-1641.

"Tallgrass Prairie Project." *Nebraska Wildlife Federation*. http://www. nebraskawildlife.org (accessed on April 17, 2007).

Tatum, Terry. "The Mystery of the Swamp Tree." *Georgia Wildlife Federation*. http:// www.gwf.org/programs/swamptree.html (accessed on July 2, 2007).

Taubes, Gary. *Good Calories, Bad Calories: Challenging the Conventional Wisdom on Diet, Weight Control, and Disease*. New York: Knopf, 2007.

----"What If It's All Been A Big Fat Lie?" *New York Times*, July 7, 2002. http:// query.nytimes.com/gst/fullpage.html?res=9F04E2D61F3EF934A35754C0A 9649C8B63 (accessed July 11, 2007).

"UN calls for strong action to eliminate violence against women." *UN News Centre.* http://www.un.org/apps/news/story.asp?NewsID=16674&Cr=&Cr1= (accessed on November 13, 2007).

Vidal, Gore. "At Home, 1988," in James A. Haught, ed., *2000 Years of Disbelief: Famous People with the Courage to Doubt.* Amherst, NY: Prometheus Books, 1996.

----*United States: Essays 1952-1992.* New York: Random House, 1993.

Voegtlin, Walter L., M.D. The Stone Age Diet. New York: Vantage Press, 1975.

Wadley, G. and A. Martin. "The Origins of Agriculture—A Biological Perspective and a New Hypothesis." *Australian Biologist,* June 1993.

Weise, Elizabeth. "World Population to Level Off." *USA Today,* December 9, 2003. http://www.usatoday.com/news/world/2003-12-09-worldpop-usat_x.htm (accessed on May 6, 2007).

"The Welfare of Sows in Gestation Crates." *Farm Sanctuary Research Report.* http://www.factoryfarming.com/pork.htm (accessed June 5, 2007).

"What is a Fruitarian?" http://www.acorn.net/fruitarian/what.html#nonviolent (accessed on February 3, 2007).

Williams, Ted. "America's River." *Audubon Magazine* 108, no. 3, May-June 2006.

----"Horse Sense." *Audubon Magazine* 108, no. 5, September-October 2006.

----"The Last Line of Defense." *Audubon Magazine* 108, no. 3, May-June 2006.

----"Wanted: More Hunters," *Audubon Magazine,* 104, no. 2, March 2002, http://www.magazine.audubon.org/incite/incite0203.html (accessed July 17, 2007).

Williams, W.L. *The Spirit and the Flesh: Sexual diversity in American Indian culture.* Boston: Beacon Press, 1992.

Wolf, Naomi. *The Beauty Myth.* New York: William Morrow and Company, Inc., 1991.

Wolfe, David. *The Sunfood Diet Success System.* San Diego: Maul Brothers Publishing, 1999.

John Yudkin. "The Causes and Cures of Obesity." *Lancet* 274, no. 7112: pp. 1135-38.

----"Diet and Coronary Thrombosis: Hypothesis and Fact." *Lancet.* 270, no. 6987: pp. 155-62.

----*Pure, White, and Deadly.* London: Davis-Poynter, 1972.

----*Sweet and Dangerous.* New York: P. H. Wyden, 1972.

----*This Slimming Business.* London: MacGibbon and Kee, 1958.

Zuriek, M. "Decline in Serum Total Cholesterol and the Risk of Death from Cancer." *Epidemiology* 8, no. 2, March 1997.

About the Author

Lierre Keith is a writer, small farmer, and radical feminist activist. She is the author of two novels and is currently co-writing a book with Derrick Jensen and Aric McBay about strategy for the environmental movement. She lives in both western Massachusetts and northern California. For upcoming appearances and events, visit her website at www.lierrekeith.com.

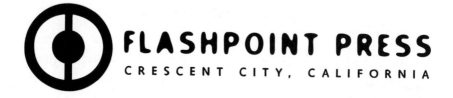

FLASHPOINT PRESS
CRESCENT CITY, CALIFORNIA

Flashpoint Press was founded by Derrick Jensen to ignite a resistance movement. Our planet is under serious threat from industrial civilization, with its consumption of biotic communities, production of greenhouse gases and environmental toxins, and destruction of human rights and human-scale cultures around the globe. This system will not stop voluntarily, and it can not be reformed.

Flashpoint Press believes that the Left has severely limited its strategic thinking, by insisting on education, lifestyle change, and techno-fixes as the only viable and ethical options. None of these responses can address the scale of the emergency now facing our planet. We need both a serious resistance movement and a supporting culture of resistance that can inspire and protect frontline activists. Flashpoint embraces the necessity of all levels of action, from cultural work to militant confrontation. We also intend to win.

Visit www.flashpointpress.com.

Special thanks to the Wallace Global Fund for their ongoing support.

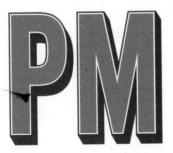

PM Press was founded at the end of 2007 by a small collection of folks with decades of publishing, media, and organizing experience. PM co-founder Ramsey Kanaan started AK Press as a young teenager in Scotland almost 30 years ago and, together with his fellow PM Press co-conspirators, has published and distributed hundreds of books, pamphlets, CDs, and DVDs. Members of PM have founded enduring book fairs, spearheaded victorious tenant organizing campaigns, and worked closely with bookstores, academic conferences, and even rock bands to deliver political and challenging ideas to all walks of life. We're old enough to know what we're doing and young enough to know what's at stake.

We seek to create radical and stimulating fiction and non-fiction books, pamphlets, t-shirts, visual and audio materials to entertain, educate and inspire you. We aim to distribute these through every available channel with every available technology - whether that means you are seeing anarchist classics at our bookfair stalls; reading our latest vegan cookbook at the café; downloading geeky fiction e-books; or digging new music and timely videos from our website.

PM Press is always on the lookout for talented and skilled volunteers, artists, activists and writers to work with. If you have a great idea for a project or can contribute in some way, please get in touch.

PM Press
PO Box 23912
Oakland, CA 94623
www.pmpress.org